Regulation of Neuroendocrine Aging

Interdisciplinary Topics in Gerontology

Vol. 24

Series Editor
H.P. von Hahn, Basel

KARGER

Basel · München · Paris · London · New York · New Delhi · Singapore · Tokyo · Sydney

Regulation of Neuroendocrine Aging

Volume Editors
Arthur V. Everitt, Sydney
Judie R. Walton, Prospect

8 figures, 1 color plate and 5 tables, 1988

KARGER

Basel · München · Paris · London · New York · New Delhi · Singapore · Tokyo · Sydney

Interdisciplinary Topics in Gerontology

Library of Congress Cataloging-in-Publication Data
Regulation of neuroendocrine aging.
(Interdisciplinary topics in gerontology; vol. 24)
Includes bibliographies and index.
1. Hypothalamic-pituitary-adrenal axis-Aging. 2. Neuroendocrinology. 3. Aging.
I. Everitt, Arthur V. II. Walton, Judie R., 1940-. III. Series.
[DNLM: 1. Aging. 2. Hormones-physiology. 3. Hypothalamo-Hypophyseal System.
Wl IN679 v. 24 / WK 502 R3435]
HQ1060.153 vol. 24 [QP188.H88] 362.6 s 88-9381 [612′.8]
ISBN 3-8055-4770-6

Drug Dosage

The authors and the publisher have exerted every effort to ensure that drug selection and dosage set forth in this text are in accord with current recommendations and practice at the time of publication. However, in view of ongoing research, changes in government regulations, and the constant flow of information relating to drug therapy and drug reactions, the reader is urged to check the package insert for each drug for any change in indications and dosage and for added warnings and precautions. This is particularly important when the recommended agent is a new and/or infrequently employed drug.

Printed in Switzerland by Thür AG, Offsetdruck, Pratteln
ISBN 3-8055-4770-6

Contents

Acknowledgements

It was a pleasure to accept the invitation of Dr. Holger von Hahn to prepare this monograph. Dr. Judie Walton kindly agreed to act as co-editor and her assistance has been invaluable. I wish to express my deepest appreciation to the authors for their splendid cooperation, to Sandra Forster, Daphne Frost and Elizabeth Stephens for secretarial assistance and to Professors Tony Broe, Keith Cairncross and Cedric Shorey for providing access to secretarial and photographic facilities.

Arthur Everitt

Foreword

The concept that hormones modulate the rate of aging has been slow to gain acceptance despite it's sensational beginning in 1889 with the rejuvenation experiments of Brown-Sequard using testicular extracts. There is now an overwhelming body of research data supporting the role of hormones in aging.

Some exciting developments during the last decade have revealed longterm damaging actions of steroid hormones on neuroendocrine regulatory neurons of the hypothalamus and hippocampus. These observations raise the possibility that hormonal feedback may not only be regulating hypothalamic-pituitary-peripheral endocrine function but simultaneously contributing to its aging. Whether these long-term actions of hormones constitute a regulation of neuroendocrine aging or represent a wear and tear breakdown of sensitive cells is controversial.

The study of regulation requires the use of experimental animals such as the rat and mouse. Human studies are limited mainly to measurement of age changes in circulating hormone levels and structural age changes in endocrine glands. Gone are the days when human data could be obtained from patients with endocrine disorders untreated for decades. Today such information can only be obtained from laboratory animals exposed to hypophysectomy, thyroidectomy, brain lesions or other operations and/or subjected to slow release hormone or neurotransmitter therapy for a large part of their life span.

This volume presents a considerable amount of experimental data showing that hormones, and nutrients with which they interact, play a major role in determining the rate of aging in most tissues of the body, including the neuroendocrine system.

November, 1987 *A.V. Everitt* and *J.R. Walton*

Interdiscipl. Topics Geront., vol. 24, pp. 1–8 (Karger, Basel 1988)

Regulation of Aging along the Hypothalamic-Pituitary-Endocrine Axis

Arthur V. Everitt[a], *Judie R. Walton*[b]

[a]Department of Geriatric Medicine, University of Sydney, Repatriation General Hospital, Concord, Australia;
[b]CSIRO Division of Animal Production, Prospect, Australia

Hormones secreted by the hypothalamic-pituitary-endocrine axis are necessary for the proper functioning of almost every cell in the body. This endocrine axis is very complex in operation, because it involves interactions with neurotransmitters of the brain, hormones produced by its different components and nutrients from the gut and liver (fig. 1). These same neurotransmitters and hormones that are concerned with the normal operation of this axis may also regulate its development in early life as well as its breakdown or aging in later life. These views have been expressed by a number of workers [1–6] (also see chapter of Segall and Sternberg in this volume) but are not accepted by all gerontologists (see chapter of Felicio and Nelson).

It must be emphasized that our knowledge of the regulation and mechanisms of neuroendocrine aging is very imperfect, even though some important discoveries have been made showing the damaging actions of hormones over long periods on certain neuroendocrine regulatory centres in the brain (see chapter of Meites). Another significant finding is that hormones may play an important role in programed cell death not only in the brain (see chapter of Segall and Sternberg) but also in the ovary and other tissues (see chapter of Goya).

Regulation of Aging

There are certain events in the life cycle that are accurately timed such as birth, puberty onset, growth cessation and menopause. All of these functions involve the actions of hormones of the hypothalamic-pituitary endo-

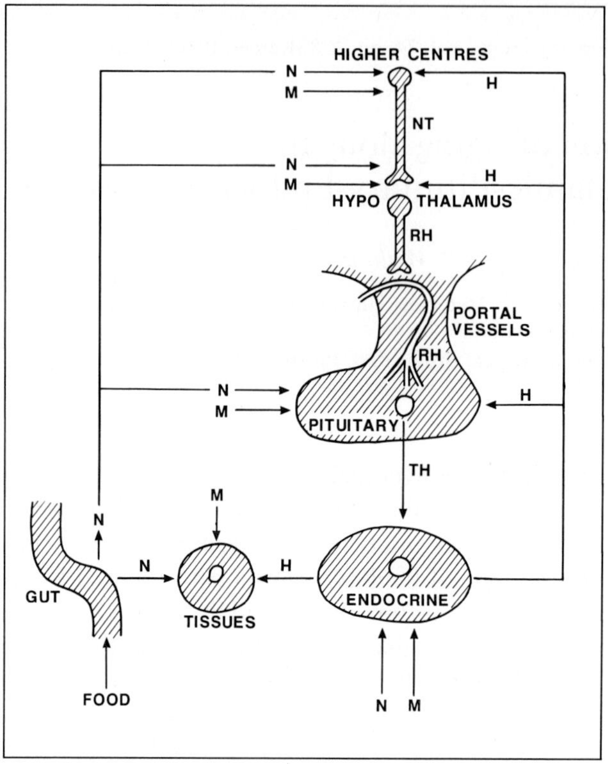

Fig. 1. Regulation of hormone secretion and aging. Information from higher centers (hippocampus, amygdala, pineal, etc.) is relayed by neurotransmitters (NT) to the hypothalamus, which secretes releasing hormones (RH) into the portal vessels to stimulate the release of pituitary tropic hormones (TH), which in turn control the secretion of hormones (H) from the peripheral endocrine glands (thyroid, adrenal cortex, gonads). Hormone secretion by the hypothalamic-pituitary-endocrine axis is regulated by the feedback of peripheral hormones (H) acting on the pituitary, hypothalamus and higher centers. Nutrients (N) absorbed from the gut act on these sites also to modulate hormone secretion. Although short-term food restriction stimulates the secretion of a number of hormones, long continued undernutrition reduces the secretion of most hormones [10] (see chapter of Merry and Holehan). The rate of aging in all tissues studied, including those of the neuroendocrine axis is retarded by dietary restriction and hypophysectomy. There is now considerable evidence to support the hypothesis that the rate of aging in the neuroendocrine axis, as in other organs, is modulated by the lifelong actions of hormones and nutrients on target tissues. The very hormones which are concerned with the normal operation of the neuroendocrine axis appear to be damaging or aging their target cells during the course of life. Hormones may affect aging by modifying gene action or by indirectly producing metabolites (M) in target tissues such as free radicals or cross-linkers which are known to accelerate aging processes.

crine axis and these events may be regulated in part by the appropriate hormones working within the confines of the genetic program.

The best evidence that aging phenomena are regulated by the hypothalamic-pituitary axis comes from lifelong studies in rodents subjected to dietary restriction, feeding of tryptophan-deficient diets or hypophysectomy (see chapters of Merry and Holehan, Segall and Sternberg, and Everitt). All three of these procedures inhibit growth and maturation as well as successfully prolonging life, retarding physiological aging and delaying the onset of age-related pathology [7–9]. Since these dietary manipulations modulate hypothalamic-pituitary function [4, 10], this provides strong evidence that the neuroendocrine system has a regulatory role in development and aging.

The most extensive research on the regulation of aging along the hypothalamic-pituitary axis has utilized the decline in reproductive function in the female rodent as a neuroendocrine model of aging. These studies reveal major species differences in the sites of the principal age defects in man, rat and mouse.

Regulation of the Reproductive Decline

In the human female the ovary is probably the primary site of the aging defect because the fall in estrogen secretion is accompanied by a compensatory rise in the production of pituitary gonadotropins and hypothalamic gonadotropin-releasing hormone (GnRH). The pituitary retains its responsiveness to GnRH in the postmenopausal woman [11].

In the old female rat the major defect is apparently at the hypothalamic level, producing a deficiency of GnRH and hence low circulating-luteinizing-hormone levels. Neuroendocrine regulation of reproductive aging in the rodent has recently been reviewed [12]. Several studies [13–15] showed that the prolonged action of estrogen from the ovary is damaging the hypothalamus, particularly the neurons of the arcuate nucleus that secrete GnRH. A reduced activity of catecholamines in the hypothalamus [16] relates to the deficient GnRH secretion. Other changes in the rat are a reduced responsiveness of the pituitary to GnRH and of the ovary to gonadotropins [6]. Age-related changes in the central cycling control precede the exhaustion of the oocyte stock in the ovary.

In the mouse changes in both the hypothalamus and ovary contribute to the reproductive decline (see chapter of Felicio and Nelson). Ovarian graft experiments in the C57BL mouse show that cessation of cycling is due to ovarian failure as in the human female, and plasma luteinizing hormone rises; increasing cycle length is due to changes in both the hypothalamic-pituitary unit and the ovary. Earlier studies had shown that the loss of oocytes from mouse ovary is affected by pituitary hormones, since the rate of loss with age is halved by hypophysectomy [17].

Testicular failure in men is gradual and the major age defect appears to be in the gonad, since blood gonadotropin levels rise while testosterone levels fall. However, in the old male rat the primary age change is probably in the hypothalamus where catecholamine levels are decreased [16]. The old male rat has low blood testosterone levels accompanied by low gonadotropin levels suggesting a central defect [18].

Regulation of the Thyroid Decline

Thyroid aging has been reviewed by several authors [19, 20]. In healthy subjects there is little or no change in plasma levels of thyroid hormones (T_3 and T_4) or thyrotropin (TSH). However, the thyroxine secretion rate is halved between age 20 and 80 and this age change is related to the loss of muscle tissue. Thus, although thyroxine is maintained in plasma at constant levels, its synthesis is apparently lowered in response to its decreased uptake and utilization by peripheral tissues. In addition to this change there is evidence of a blunted TSH response to thyrotropin-releasing hormone. Serum T_3 may be lower in the aged due to reduced deiodination of T_4 to T_3.

Most studies in the rat show age decrements in plasma T_4 and T_3, and an increased conversion of T_4 to T_3 in tissues in old age is reported. There is no compensatory rise in TSH in female rats, although it has been observed in males. A fall in the secretion of hypothalamic thyrotropin-releasing hormone in the old rat [21] may contribute to the fall in thyroid hormone secretion.

Regulation of Adrenocortical Aging

Adrenocortical aging is discussed by several workers [22, 23]. In healthy human subjects hypothalamic-pituitary-adrenocortical function is normal in old age permitting the individual to withstand moderate stress.

Although basal plasma cortisol levels do not change in elderly subjects, there is a 25% decrease in their 24-hour cortisol secretion compared with younger subjects. This decrement relates to the slower metabolism of cortisol in old age.

In aging rats most reports indicate that both basal and stress-induced levels of blood glucocorticoids rise with age [24], probably due to increased adrenocorticotropic hormone secretion [25]. Glucocorticoids and stress accelerate morphological age changes and loss of glucocorticoid receptors in the hippocampus and such changes may contribute to the elevated adrenocorticotropic hormone and glucocorticoid secretion [22, 24] in old age (see chapter of Sharma and Timiras). Food restriction and hypophysectomy slow accumulation of age pigments in rat adrenal cortex (see chapter of Walton et al.).

Regulation of Growth Hormone Decline

Growth hormone (GH) changes with age are discussed in detail in the chapter of Sonntag and Meites. GH pulsatile secretion is decreased during sleep in elderly human subjects [26] and this is associated with a decline in somatomedin C levels [27]. In women pulsatile secretion may be amplified by estradiol [28]. There is also a decrease in the pulsatile secretion in old rats [29]. It has been suggested [6] that a decline in hypothalamic norepinephrine activity in old rats increases somatostatin production which inhibits GH secretion. Since GH enhances protein synthesis, diminished GH secretion in old age may contribute to the loss of lean body mass, including bone.

Regulation of Prolactin Aging

Prolactin (PRL) secretion in men shows no change with age, however, decrements are seen in postmenopausal women in relation to the declining estrogen secretion [30]. In both sexes of the old rat PRL secretion increases with age in association with the development of PRL-secreting tumors of the pituitary [13, 31]. The age defect in the rat appears to be a degeneration of dopaminergic neurons, thereby reducing hypothalamic dopamine secretion and elevating pituitary PRL secretion [31]. Damage to dopaminergic neurons may be caused by chronic exposure to PRL or estrogen which stimulates PRL secretion [6].

Regulation of Neurohypophyseal Aging

In the rat the secretion of the vasopressin appears to decrease in old age (chapter of Zbuzek and Zbuzek), although the age change in man is not clear. Whether the decrement in vasopressin secretion is due to changes in central regulation by neurotransmitters or by other mechanisms is unknown.

Rejuvenation Studies

Between 1889 and 1925 the rejuvenation studies of Brown-Sequard, Voronoff and Steinach unsuccessfully attempted to revive failing testicular function in human subjects. In recent years with a better understanding of the neuroendocrine and immunological factors in aging rejuvenation research is on a sounder basis. Most current rejuvenation studies using hormones, neurotransmitters and neuron transplants are concerned with elucidating regulatory mechanisms of aging, but they also have practical implications. The chapters of Peng et al and Huang describe work using neurotransmitters in slow release capsules or hypothalamic grafts, both of which improved sex functions in old rats. We can expect that rejuvenation techniques will be applicable to human beings in the foreseeable future.

Aging Regulatory Centers

The hypothalamic-pituitary-endocrine axis is a self-regulating system with hypothalamic centers receiving feedback of hormones from the peripheral endocrine glands (thyroid, adrenal cortex, gonads). Does this system continue to function normally until some components wear out due to long-continued action of hormones or other agents (free radicals, neurotransmitters, food factors, etc.) on its target cells (fig. 1)? Or is aging in this system a regulated phenomenon, in which the breakdown involving hormonal action on a target is programed? The fact that the sites of breakdown are characteristic for the species and the age when lesions develop are more or less fixed lends support to the regulated program theory. The idea of a clock in the hypothalamus [1] timing the rate of aging by controlling the secretion of aging hormones has been questioned by Finch et al.

[15] whose studies have shown that there is not a fixed number of estrous cycles in the rodent before the failure of reproduction. Even if the hypothalamus does not have a direct timing role in aging, it certainly controls the secretion of all hormones by the neuroendocrine system and by the actions of these hormones probably influences the rate of aging in the whole hypothalamic-pituitary-endocrine axis.

References

1 Everitt, A.V.: The hypothalamic-pituitary control of aging and age-related pathology. Exp. Gerontol. *8:* 265–277 (1973).
2 Denckla, W.A.: A time to die. Life Sci. *16:* 31–44 (1975).
3 Finch, C.E.: The regulation of physiological changes during mammalian aging. Q. Rev. Biol. *51:* 49–83 (1976).
4 Segall, P.E.: Interrelations of dietary and hormonal effects in aging. Mech. Age. Dev. *9:* 515–525 (1979).
5 Timiras, P.S.; Choy, V.J.; Hudson, D.B.: Neuroendocrine pacemaker for growth, development and ageing. Age Ageing *11:* 73–88 (1982).
6 Meites, J.; Goya, R.; Takahashi, S.: Why the neuroendocrine system is important in aging processes. Exp. Gerontol. *22:* 1–15 (1987).
7 Holehan, A.M.; Merry, B.J.: The experimental manipulation of ageing by diet. Biol. Rev. *61:* 329–368 (1986).
8 Segall, P.E.; Timiras, P.S.; Walton, J.R.: Low tryptophan diets delay reproductive aging. Mech. Age. Dev. *23:* 245–252 (1983).
9 Everitt, A.V.; Seedsman, N.J.; Jones, F.: The effects of hypophysectomy and continuous food restriction, begun at ages 70 and 400 days, on collagen aging, proteinuria, incidence of pathology and longevity in the male rat. Mech. Age. Dev. *12:* 161–172 (1980).
10 Everitt, A.V.; Porter, B.: Nutrition and aging; in Everitt, Burgess, Hypothalamus, pituitary and aging, pp. 570–613 (Thomas, Springfield 1976).
11 DeKretser, D.M.; Burger, H.G.; Dumpys, R.: Patterns of serum LH and FSH in response to 4 hour infusions of LHRH in normal women during the menstrual cycle on oral contraceptives and in postmenopausal state. J. clin. Endocr. Metab. *46:* 227–235 (1978).
12 Cooper, R.L.; Goldman, J.M.; Rehnberg, G.L.: Neuroendocrine control of reproductive function in the aging female rodent. J. Am. Geriat. Soc. *34:* 735–751 (1986).
13 Aschheim, P.: Aging in the hypothalamic-hypophyseal-ovarian axis in the rat; in Everitt, Burgess, Hypothalamus, pituitary and aging, pp. 376–418 (Thomas, Springfield 1976).
14 Brawer, J.R.; Schipper, H.; Naftolin, F.: Ovary-dependent degeneration in the hypothalamic arcuate nucleus. Endocrinology *107:* 274–279 (1980).
15 Finch, C.E.; Felicio, L.S.; Mobbs, C.V.; Nelson, J.F.: Ovarian and steroidal influences on neuroendocrine aging processes in female rodents. Endocr. Rev. *5:* 467–497 (1984).

16 Simpkins, J.W.: Mueller, G.P.; Huang, H.H.; Meites, J.: Evidence for depressed catecholamine and enhanced serotonin metabolism in aging male rats: possible relation to gonadotropin secretion. Endocrinology *100:* 1672–1678 (1977).
17 Jones, E.C.; Krohn, P.L.: The effect of hypophysectomy on age changes in the ovaries of mice. J. Endocr. *21:* 497–509 (1961).
18 Riegle, G.D.: Endocrine regulation of the testis in the aged male; in Adelman, Roth, Endocrine and neuroendocrine mechanisms of aging, pp. 105–121 (CRC Press, Boca Raton 1982).
19 Gregerman, R.I.: Regulation of thyrotropin physiology during aging; in Meites, Neuroendocrinology of aging, pp. 259–274 (Plenum Press, New York 1983).
20 Gambert, S.R.; Tsitouras, P.D.: Effect of age on thyroid hormone physiology and function. J. Am. Geriat. Soc. *33:* 360–365 (1985).
21 Peckary, A.E.; Mirrell, C.J.; Turner, L.F.; Walfish, P.G.; Horshman, J.M.: Hypothalamic secretion of thyrotropin releasing hormone declines in old rats. J. Geront. *42:* 447–450 (1987).
22 Sapolsky, R.M.; Krey, L.C.; McEwen, B.S.: The neuroendocrinology of stress and aging. The glucocorticoid cascade hypothesis. Endocr. Rev. *7:* 284–301 (1986).
23 Everitt, A.V.; Andrews, G.R.: Hypothalamo-hypophyseal-adrenal axis; in Platt, Geriatrics 2, pp. 88–101 (Springer, Berlin 1983).
24 Landfield, P.; Waymire, J.; Lynch, G.: Hippocampal aging and adrenocorticoids: a quantitative correlation. Science *202:* 1098–1102 (1978).
25 Tang, F.; Phillips, J.G.: Some age-related changes in pituitary-adrenal function in the male laboratory rat. J. Geront. *33:* 377–382 (1978).
26 Finkelstein, J.W.: Roffwarg, H.P.; Boyar, R.M.; Kream, J.; Hellman, L.: Age-related change in the twenty-four-hour spontaneous secretion of growth hormone. J. clin. Endocr. *35:* 665–670 (1972).
27 Florini, J.R.; Prinz, P.N.; Vitiello, M.V.; Hintz, R.L.: Somatomedin-C levels in healthy young and old men: relationship to peak and 24 hour integrated levels of growth hormone. J. Geront. *40:* 2–7 (1985).
28 Ho, K.Y.; Evans, W.S.; Blizzard, R.M.; Veldhuis, J.D.; Merriam, G.R.; Samojlik, E.; Furlanetto, R.; Rogol, A.D.; Kaiser, D.L.; Thorner, M.O.: Effects of sex and age on the 24-hour profile of growth hormone secretion in man: importance of endogenous estradiol concentrations. J. clin. Endocr. Metab. *64:* 51–58 (1987).
29 Sonntag, W.E.; Steger, R.W.; Forman, L.J.; Meites, J.: Decreased pulsatile release of growth hormone in old male rats. Endocrinology *107:* 1875–1879 (1980).
30 Bulbrook, R.D.; Wang, D.Y.; Hayward, J.L.; Kwa, H.G.; Cleton, F.: Plasma prolactin levels and age in a female population: relation to breast cancer. Int. J. Cancer *28:* 43–45 (1981).
31 Gudelsky, G.A.; Nansel, D.D.; Porter, J.C.: Dopaminergic control of prolactin secretion in the aging male rat. Brain Res. *204:* 446–450 (1981).

Dr. A.V. Everitt, Department of Geriatric Medicine, Ward 29, Concord Hospital, Concord, NSW 2139 (Australia)

Interdiscipl. Topics Geront., vol. 24, pp. 9–20 (Karger, Basel 1988)

Aging: A CNS-Endocrine Perspective

Paul E. Segall, Hal Sternberg

Department of Physiology-Anatomy, University of California at Berkeley, Berkeley, Calif., USA

To say that there is disagreement among gerontologists regarding the mechanisms underlying aging is to understate the issue. Indeed, there may be as many theories of aging as there are those who study it. Rather than briefly categorizing each of the published theories, which involve the neuroendocrine sytem, let us focus on a few approaches currently favored by some active laboratories in the field. There are several reviews to which one may refer for a more comprehensive survey of the question [1–3].

It is possible, to some extent, to group neuroendocrine theories of aging. One viewpoint proposes that aging originates from a loss of program associated with progressive dysfunction in neuroendocrine command cell populations [1]. Several possible sources of such disruptive effects can be cited, e.g. (a) ionizing radiation [4, 5] which jeopardizes the cell's genetic material, (b) cross-linking agents [6] thought to place 'molecular handcuffs' on intracellular components such as the genetic material and its companion nucleoprotein, and (c) highly reactive oxidative free radicals [7], which may alter informational macromolecules, form insoluble, accumulating precipitates, and alter intracellular membranes [8].

Free Radical Oxidative Damage

Especially interesting is the proposition that one class of neuron which seems to be compromised by aging, the catecholaminergics [2, 9–11], generates relatively high levels of potentially destructive oxidative free radicals. The importance of catecholaminergic neurons in neuroendocrine function is unchallenged. They have been implicated in the control of a variety of hypothalamic neuroendocrine activities, including the luteinizing hormone [11–13], the secretion of growth hormone [14], and the inhibition of prolactin release [15–17].

Can aging be caused by an accumulation of damage due to oxidative free radicals [8, 18]? It is well known that all neurons are very active in their uptake and utilization of oxygen. The 'aging pigments' characteristic of neurons and endocrine cells are thought by some to be the nondigestable waste products of oxidative metabolism [19, 20]. Both the CNS, and the endocrines which they regulate are central players in governing a wide variety of physiological processes and the tissues in which these processes reside. Events which damage the brain and the endocrines must impair those body activities and structures under their control.

Hormonal Damage

An alternative view of neuroendocrine aging postulates that high levels of certain hormones, especially steroids, can lead to the loss of brain cells, processes, or synapses, to which they feed back and bind [21–26]. There is some evidence that this occurs in the medial basal hypothalamus [24–27] as well as in the hippocampus of some animals [21, 22]. Along with the loss of such neurons or synapses is the loss of their function. Since their function can be the downregulation of the secretion of the steroid at fault, a positive feedback phenomenon may ensue, driving steroid levels upward. Not only could the resulting high steroid levels further damage susceptible neurons, these elevated levels may also have negative effects on nonneural tissues, such as those of the immunological system. The body is thus rendered less able to defend against age-related morbid processes such as cancer [21].

Programed Neuroendocrine Effects

It is becoming widely recognized that the development of the vertebrate [28, 29] and mammalian [30] nervous system involves a considerable amount of programed cell death. Programed cell death may play a role in maturation as well. There is evidence that loss of cells, or at least interruption of their activities, is crucial in the 'resetting' of the hypothalamus during puberty. Lesioning the area between the anterior and medial basal hypothalamus has been shown experimentally to induce precocious puberty [31], suggesting that some of the neurons whose processes were interrupted may have been inhibitory to the medial basal region, to which they normally connect.

There are a number of competing ideas about what happens in the hypothalamus to cause puberty [32]. One hypothesis based on lesioning experiments states that just prior to puberty, a group of cells in the anterior hypothalamus die. Throughout the juvenile period, this cell population inhibits the medial basal hypothalamus.

The loss of members of this inhibitory cell population during maturation disinhibits the medial basal hypothalamus, allowing increased lutein-releasing-hormone production and release, stimulating pituitary gonadotropic activity, and consequently, initiating gonadal steroid secretion. These gonadal steroids then feed back, bind to, and kill the above inhibitory neurons which bear steroid receptors. An explosive release of gonadal steroids occur, resulting in sexual maturation.

When neurons, their processes, or their synapses are lost, other neurons in contact with those lost or attenuated may be affected. One programed perspective on neuroendocrine aging suggests that such predetermined specific cell population losses may set off a cascade of cell population losses and inactivations. This progressive cascade of cell death and loss of function, inextricably tied to maturation, may be ultimately responsible for much of what is usually found during aging. To summarize, initial developmental losses engender further maturational losses, which in turn underlie subsequent losses leading to senescence [33].

There are other examples of such cell population losses during maturation. The substantial loss of egg cells from the female mammalian ovary is a familiar example of maturation-related cell death occurring throughout the juvenile period [34]. The shrinking of the thymus following maturation is yet another [35].

The same dynamics may underlie maturation and aging of the spinal cord and the autonomic nervous system. Can their aging be tied to maturational events during which populations of CNS neurons become lost or nonfunctional? Can cascades of cell population losses and inactivations which accompany aging be linked to such maturational events? The answers to these questions may tell much about aging, and allow the development of more effective ways to clinically intervene in its unpleasant consequences.

Neuroendocrine Effects of Dietary Restriction

Delayed aging due to dietary restriction has called attention to the role of neuroendocrine phenomena in gerontological processes. Female rats, fed low tryptophan diets starting at early weaning, and then fed normally 12–29 months later [36, 37], have been shown to produce and nurture young at ages when more than 90% of untreated controls have died of age-related pathology. Calorie-restricted female rats also show fecundity at ages up to 29 months [38]. As the importance of the neuroendocrine system is well established in the development and regulation of the reproductive function, there can be no doubt that nutritional restriction, the most effective and possibly only reliably known method of slowing aging in mammals, has a key effect on the neuroendocrine system.

Since underfeeding is so effective in retarding the aging process, it may be useful to examine its impact from the perspective of the above neuroendocrine theories. One could argue that nutritional restriction retards aging by slowing the metabolic generation of oxidative free radicals, or by stimulating and enhancing protective mechanisms thought to neutralize their destructiveness.

There are a number of problems with this approach. Firstly, it has not been proven that nutritional restriction slows the generation of free radicals. A number of studies aimed at this question have failed to conclusively demonstrate that nutritional restriction actually lowers the rate of oxygen consumption per unit animal tissue; in some cases, underfeeding raises it [38, 39]. Recently, there is some evidence [40] from mouse studies that nutritional restriction raises levels of liver catalase, an enzyme which can protect tissue against hydrogen peroxide. However, this has yet to be shown in the brain. Furthermore, even if this appears to be the case, this rise may only be to compensate other protective systems negatively impacted by nutritional restriction.

A more powerful criticism emerges from experiments utilizing nutritional restriction initiated at weaning, and at ages later than weaning. Experiments indicate that rodents placed on restricted diets very early in life exhibit remarkably extended lifespans, in some cases beyond 1,500 days [41], 1,600 days [42], 1,700 days [43] and even 1,800 days [44]. Studies, in which these diets are initiated later, such as 6 weeks of age [45], 70 days of age [46], and 6 months of age [45] show life spans extended, but not much beyond 1,300 days [45, 46]. While it is true that these latter animals live substantially longer than controls, oxidative damage alone operating for a few more weeks can hardly explain why rats placed on restricted diets a little later in life do not show maximum life spans of 1,600–1,800 days.

Hormone toxicity theories, however, can explain this phenomenon quite readily. Nutritional restriction has been likened in some ways to a 'nutritional hypophysectomy' [47]. Underfeeding can alter levels of pituitary hormones, as well as those from their target organs [38]. Indeed, retardation of aging has also been reported in hypophysectomized animals [46]. One interpretation of delayed aging in underfed rats is that nutritional restriction simply lowers the circulating quantities of steroids. Reduced levels of steroids spare cell populations normally destroyed by these hormones. The earlier the hypophysectomy, or the beginning of the restriction, the more cells are spared from 'feedback death'. If there are populations of cells particularly sensitive to these hormones prior to puberty, nutritional restriction initiated at weaning will protect these cells from high steroid titers. If the restriction is started later, then a number of these cells may be lost.

The total amount of 17β-estradiol and progesterone released by food-restricted females has been shown to be reduced. Dietary restriction can also suppress the stress-related rise of corticosterone in postweaning rats, although by 1 year of age this effect could no longer be observed [38]. If high levels of these steroids are cytotoxic to hypothalamic neurons which bind them, nutritionally restricted animals may be somewhat protected from steroid damage suspected in controls. This could explain some aspects of their retarded reproductive aging.

Undernutrition Delays Cell Death

Another possible explanation of the antiaging effects of undernutrition is its potential impact on cell death throughout the neuroendocrine system, and even on other systems influenced by the brain and the endocrines, such as the immune system [35]. Interference with programed cell death may account for the delay in reproductive maturation and aging seen when young female Long-Evans rats are fed diets low in tryptophan for extended periods [36].

When rats were fed low tryptophan diets from 3 weeks of age, a few of the rats severely deprived (fed on a diet containing 30% of the tryptophan content of controls) were able to reproduce at 30 months or beyond, once they were returned to a normal diet. However, rats fed on a slightly less deprived diet, one containing 40% of the tryptophan content of controls [36], or fed very low tryptophan diets starting at 3 months of age [37], could not reproduce at late ages.

The growth of rats fed on low tryptophan diets from weaning is related to the amount of tryptophan in the diet 48], as is the amount of food consumed daily [41]. Slow growth in animals fed diets low in tryptophan may be due to the lack of this essential amino acid needed for protein formation. The decline noted in the rate of food intake of these animals [41, 49] suggests the action of regulatory mechanisms which perceive the lack of tryptophan and globally downregulate protein synthesis.

The fecal pellets of rats fed diets containing the lowest levels of tryptophan are pale in color compared to those of rats fed the same diet with tryptophan added back in normal amounts [50]. Color of fecal pellets comes from bile pigments emptied into the intestine. Bile pigments derive from the breakdown of hemoglobin. Under conditions of reduced protein intake, protein synthesis, and thus certain forms of cell replication which depend on it, may diminish. Therefore, red blood cell production may be suppressed in rats fed the low tryptophan diet. The organism, sensing the lack of both a cellular building block (tryptophan) and energy (calories), may reduce its rate of erythropoiesis.

The organism may also reduce its rate of cell loss, and therefore the amount of hemoglobin breakdown products in the blood. Low concentrations of these hemoglobin breakdown products in the blood would lessen their presence in the bile, and therefore in the intestine. Fecal color would thus be lightened.

Reduced DNA synthesis, as measured by in vivo incorporation of ^{3}H thymidine, was recorded in liver, heart, kidney and abdominal skin, but not in thymus and small intestine, of food-restricted animals [38], suggesting that underfeeding halted cell proliferation in many (but not all) tissues. Evidence is mounting that along with cell proliferation, dietary restriction also slows cell death.

Intact and functionally appearing ovarian follicles observed in 3-year-old rats fed low tryptophan diets for 2 years or more illustrate the retarded cell loss seen in rats maintained on very low tryptophan diets from weaning until late ages [48]. Reduced rates of egg cell loss have been reported previously in rats fed from weaning on low tryptophan [36] or calorie-restricted diets [51]. Rats fed on low tryptophan diets have incubated fully formed fetuses at ages approaching 3 years, illustrating that this form of nutritional restriction can preserve at least some viable oocytes for this length of time.

Other examples of retarded cell loss in dietary restriction have been reported in pinealocytes [52] and in corneal cells [53]. The rapid involution of thymus tissue seen in 100-day-old control animals was not found in food-restricted rats [38]. It is possible that the delay seen in the aging process of nutritionally deprived rats depends on the slowing of the loss of specific cell populations. In fact, aging itself may depend upon a cascade of such specific cell population losses.

There is behavioral evidence that underfeeding can affect the brain [37]. Since serotonin levels in three different specific brain regions were lower in low-tryptophan-fed rats after the implementation of the diets [48, 54], and higher after calorie restriction [41, 54], it is clear that a variety of underfeeding protocols can affect the brain.

Brain Cell Death in Development and Aging

One mechanism for the onset of puberty may be the preprogramed loss of these inhibitory neurons. If a severe nutritional restriction, either by means of a low tryptophan or low calorie diet is implemented early, this preprogramed loss of inhibitory neurons may be delayed. Perhaps the restricted diet signals the body and brain that since there is a scarcity of energy and building blocks for cell proliferation, cell loss is likewise not acceptable. Reproductive maturation, and also reproductive aging, may then be delayed as a consequence.

During the course of normal maturation, such a loss of inhibitory neurons in the hypothalamus may ultimately engender a secondary loss in neural populations either receiving impulses from or sending impulses to them. This secondary loss could result in a tertiary set of losses, thus creating a cascade of specific nerve cell loss.

It has been shown that neurons are lost in the anterior and medial preoptic nuclei of female [55], but not male [56] rats during aging. Cascading hypothalamic neuronal losses originating both as a consequence of developmentally programed losses of nerve cells and periodic peaks in estrogen levels during the estrus cycle may result in the aging of the hypothalamic areas governing reproduction, and thus causing reproductive senescence. In rats fed low tryptophan diets, or restricted in calories at early ages, both maturational nerve cell loss and high levels of estrogen may be avoided. This may explain why reproductive aging is delayed in such animals.

Specific nerve cell population losses, leading to a cascade of secondary neuronal loss and inactivation [28, 29], as well as somatic effects creating even further deleterious consequences, may account for the aging of other brain functions, and aging in other physiological systems [57]. *Severe* nutritional restriction, started *early,* may delay or prevent such losses, and this may be the origin of the ability of underfeeding to delay aging. The earlier and more severe the underfeeding, the more completely this cascade of cell loss and inactivation may be blocked.

The high juvenile mortality of animals placed on severe low-tryptophan diets appears to be due to individual variation within the strain, as maximal age-retarding effects, such as delayed reproductive aging and extended longevity, are achieved at levels of tryptophan deficiency which permit only the most minimal growth of some rats; others, due to individual differences, lose weight and die prematurely on the same diet [48]. If the diets were custom-implemented for each animal so they could eat enough to support a minimal growth rate, early mortality may be abolished, and even greater maximum life span and extended fecundity might be observed.

Developmentally Scheduled Regression of the Reproductive Hypothalamus as a Model for Aging

Is there a path which may lead to a comprehensive understanding of the role of the nervous and endocrine systems in aging? An understanding of specific cell population changes in particular brain areas from weaning, through the juvenile period, puberty and maturation, and into senescence, may reveal just such information.

Examining reproductive aging in the female rodent may be the most effective way to develop an understanding of the mechanisms underlying aging. Reproductive aging is relatively quick in rats and mice, senescent changes in cyclicity and structures becoming detectable within the 1st year of life [27, 51]. In mice, specific nuclei within the hypothalamus can be identified which contain as little as several hundred cells.

The integration of neuroanatomical, enzymatic, histochemical and molecular biological data from specific nuclei of the anterior and medial basal hypothalamus accumulated over the reproductive life span of the female rodent should provide a sophisticated understanding of the role of the brain in reproductive senescence, and how changes during the juvenile, pubertal and adult stages contribute to reproductive failure. Since nutritional restriction can delay reproductive aging, comparing changes in the anterior and medial basal hypothalamic neuronal populations of the normal and food-restricted female rodent should reveal much of how underfeeding retards reproductive aging. A vivid understanding of reproductive senescence should then shed light on the overall process of aging itself.

References

1 Meites, J.; Goya, R.; Takahashi, S.: Why the neuroendocrine system is important in aging processes. Exp. Gerontol. *22:* 1–5 (1987).

2 Timiras, P.S.: Neuroendocrinology of aging; in Meites, Neuroendocrinology of aging, pp. 5–30 (Plenum Press, New York 1983).

3 Everitt, A.V.: The genetic clock-hormone theory of aging; in Preston, Biological and social aspects of mortality and length of life, pp. 279–301 (Ordina, Liège 1982).

4 Curtis, H.J.: Biological mechanisms underlying the aging process. Science *141:* 686–694 (1963).

5 Yielding, E.L.: A model for aging based on differential repair of somatic mutational damage. Perspect. Biol. Med. *17:* 210 (1974).

6 Von Hahn, H.P.; Fritz, E.: Age-related alterations in the structure of DNA. III. Thermal stability of rat liver DNA, related to age, histone content and ionic strength. Gerontologia *12:* 237 (1966).

7 Harman, D.: The free radical theory of aging; in Prior, Free radicals in biology, vol. 5, pp. 255–275 (Pryor, Academic Press, New York 1982).

8 Melhorn, R.J.; Cole, G.: The free radical theory of aging: a critical review. Adv. Free radical Biol. Med. *1:* 165–223 (1985).

9 McNeil, T.H.; Koek, L.L.: Age-correlated changes in dopaminergic nigrostriatal perikarya of the $C_{57}BL/6$ NN_{ia} mouse. Mech. Age. Dev. *24:* 293–301 (1984).

10 Simpkins, J.W.: Regional changes in monoamine metabolism in the aging constant estrous rat. Neurobiol. Aging *5:* 309–312 (1984).

11 Walker, R.F.: Impact of age-related changes in serotonin and norepinephrine metabolism on reproductive function in female rats: an analytical review. Neurobiol. Aging *5:* 121–141 (1984).

12 Wise, P.M.: Comments on the role of monoamines, particularly serotonin in aging. Neurobiol. Aging *5:* 142–143 (1984).

13 Meites, J.: Comments on review by Dr. Richard F. Walker: relative roles of noradrenergic and serotonergic systems. Neurobiol. Aging *5:* 140–141 (1984).

14 Sonntag, W.E.; Forman, L.J.; Meites, J.: Changes in growth hormone secretion in aging rats and man, and possible relation to diminished physiological function; in Meites, Neuroendocrinology of aging, pp. 275–308 (Plenum Press, New York 1983).

15 Sarkar, D.K.; Gottschall, P.E.; Meites, J.: Relation of the neuroendocrine system to development of prolactin-secreting pituitary tumors; in Meites, Neuroendocrinology of aging, pp. 353–376 (Plenum Press, New York 1983).
16 Sarkar, D.K.; Gottschall, P.E.; Meites, J.: Damage to hypothalamic dopaminergic neurons is associated with development of prolactin-secreting pituitary tumors. Science *218:* 684–686 (1982).
17 Sarkar, D.K.; Gottschall, P.E.; Meites, J.: Relation of hypothalamic biogenic amines to secretion of gonadotropins and prolactin in the aging rat; in Cherkin, et al., Physiology and cell biology of aging, pp. 87–94 (Raven Press, New York 1979).
18 Harman, D.: The aging process. Proc. natn. Acad. Sci. *78:* 7124–7128 (1981).
19 Sohal, R.S.: In age pigments (Elsevier/North Holland Biomedical Press, Amsterdam 1981).
20 Tappel, A.: Effect of antioxidants and nutrients on lipid peroxidation fluorescent products and aging parameters in the mouse. J. Geront. *28:* 415–424 (1973).
21 Sapolsky, R.M.; Kery, L.C.; McEwen, B.S.: The neuroendocrinology of stress and aging. The glucocorticoid cascade hypothesis. Endocr. Rev. *7:* 284–301 (1986).
22 Sapolsky, R.M.; Kery, L.C.; McEwen, B.S.: Prolonged glucocorticoid exposure reduces hippocampal neuron number: implications for aging. J. Neurosci. *5:* 1221–1227 (1985).
23 Sapolsky, R.M.: A mechanism for glucocorticoid toxicity in the hippocampus: increased neural vulnerability to metabolic insults. J. Neurosci. *5:* 1228–1232 (1985).
24 Finch, C.E.: Landfield, P.W.: Neuroendocrine and autonomic function in aging mammals; in Finch, Schneider, Handbook of the biology of aging, pp. 567–594 (Van Nostrand & Reinhold, New York 1985).
25 Brawer, J.R.; Finch, C.E.: Normal and experimentally altered aging processes in the rodent hypothalamus and pituitary; in Walker, Cooper, Experimental and clinical interventions in aging. pp. 45–65 (Dekker, New York 1983).
26 Finch, C.E.; Mobbs, C.V.: Hormonal influences on hypothalamic sensitivity during aging in female rodents; in Meites, Neuroendocrinology of aging, pp. 143–171 (Plenum Press, New York 1983).
27 Finch, C.E.; Felicia, L.S.; Mobbs, C.V.; Nelson, J.F.: Ovarian and steroidal influences on neuroendocrine aging processes in female rodents. Endocr. Rev. *5:* 467–497 (1984).
28 Fahrbach, S.E.; Truman, J.W.: Mechanisms for programmed cell death in the nervous system of a moth; in Selective neuronal death. Ciba Fdn Symp. *126:* 65–81 (1987).
29 Hamburger, V.; Oppenheim, R.W.: Naturally occurring neuronal death in vertebrates. Neurosci. Comment. *1:* 39–55 (1982).
30 Comans, P.E.; McLennan, I.S.; Mark, R.F.: Mammalian motoneuron cell death: development of the lateral motor column of a wallaby *(Macripus eugenii).* J. comp. Neurol. *260:* 627–634 (1987).
31 Sherwood, N.M.; Timiras, P.S.: Comparison of direct-current and radiofrequency lesions in the rostral hypothalamus with respect of sexual maturation in the female rat. Endocrinology *9:* 1275–1286 (1974).
32 Ramalay, J.A.; The neuroendocrinology of puberty; in Vernadakis, Timiras, Hormones in development and aging, pp. 305–329 (Spectrum, New York 1982).

33 Segall, P.E.: Aging as a programmed cascade of specific cell death. Age *7:* 149 (1984).

34 Talbert, G.B.: Aging of the reproductive system; in Finch, Hayflick, The handbook of the biology of aging, chap. 13 (Van Nostrand & Reinhold, New York 1977).

35 Cross, R.J.; Markesbery, W.R.; Brooks, W.H.; Roszman, T.L.: Hypothalamic-immune interactions. I. The acute effect of anterior hypothalamic lesions on the immune response. Brain Res. *196:* 79–87 (1980).

36 Segall, P.E.; Timiras, P.S.; Walton, J.R.: Low tryptophan diets delay reproductive aging. Mech. Age. Dev. *23:* 245–252 (1983).

37 Segall, P.E.; Timiras, P.S.: Pathophysiologic findings after chronic tryptophan deficiency in rats. A model for delayed growth and aging. Mech. Age. Dev. *5:* 109–124 (1976).

38 Holehan, A.M.; Merry, B.J.: Experimental manipulation of aging by diet; in Timiras, Physiology of aging. chap. 25 (MacMillan, New York, 1987, in press).

39 McCarter, R.; Masoro, E.J.; Yee, B.P.: Does food restriction retard aging by reducing the metabolic rate? Am. J. Physiol. *248:* E488–E490 (1985).

40 Koizumi, A.; Weindruch, R.; Walford, R.L.: Influence of dietary restriction and age on liver enzyme activities and lipid peroxidation in mice. J. Nutr. *117:* 361–367 (1987).

41 Timiras, P.S.; Hudson, D.B.; Segall, P.E.: Lifetime brain serotonin: regional effects of age and precursor availability. Neurobiol. Aging *5:* 235–242 (1984).

42 Weindruch, R.; Walford, R.L.; Fligiel, S.; Guthrie, D.: The retardation of aging in mice by dietary restriction: longevity, cancer, immunity and lifetime energy intake. J. Nutr. *116:* 641–654 (1986).

43 Harrison, D.E.; Archer, J.R.: Genetic differences in effects of food restriction on aging in mice. J. Nutr. *117:* 376–382 (1987).

44 Ross, M.H.: Nutrition and longevity in experimental animals; in Winick, Nutrition and aging, pp. 43–57 (Wiley, New York 1976).

45 Yu, B.P.; Masoro, E.J.; McMahan, C.A.: Nutritional influences on aging of Fischer 344 rats: physical, metabolic, and longevity characteristcis. J. Geront. *40:* 657–670 (1985).

46 Everitt, A.V.; Seedsman, N.J.; Jones, F.: The effects of hypophysectomy and continuous food restriction, begun at ages 70 and 400 days, on collagen aging, proteinurea, incidence of pathology and longevity in the male rat. Mech. Age. Dev. *12:* 161–172 (1980).

47 Everitt, A.V.; Porter, B.: Nutrition and aging; in Everitt, Burgess, Hypothalamus, pituitary and aging, chap. 13, pp. 570–613 (Thomas, Springfield 1976).

48 Ooka, H.; Segall, P.E.; Timiras, P.S.: Histology and survival in age-delayed low-tryptophan-fed rats. Mech. Age. Dev. (submitted, 1987).

49 Ooka, H.; Segall, P.E.; Timiras, P.S.: Neural and endocrine development after chronic tryptophan deficiency in rats. II. Pituitary-thyroid axis. Mech. Age. Dev. *7:* 19–24 (1978).

50 Bellport, V.; Steinberg, R.; Young, G.W.; Ranganatham, S.; Sternberg, H.; Segall, P.E.: Timiras, P.S.: Maturational changes in regional hypothalamic neurochemistry of tryptophan-restricted rats. 71st Annu. Meet. Fed. Am. Soc. Exp. Biol., Washington 1987).

51 Nelson, J.; Goschen, R.; Felicio, L.: Effect of dietary restriction on estrous cyclicity and follicular reserves in aging C57 BL/6J mice. Biol. Reprod. *32:* 515–522 (1985).
52 Walker, R.F.; McMahon, K.M.; Pivorun, E.B.: Pineal gland structure and respiration as affected by age and hypocaloric diet. Exp. Gerontol. *13:* 91–99 (1978).
53 Nadakavukaren, M.J.; Fitch, K.L.; Richardson, A.: Rat corneal epithelial cells as markers of physiological age: dietary restriction retards age-related increase in cell area. Gerontologist *26:* 157A (1986).
54 Segall, P.E.; Ooka, H.; Rose, K.; Timiras, P.S.: Neural and endocrine development after chronic tryptophan deficiency in rats. I. Brain monoamine and pituitary responses. Mech. Age. Dev. *7:* 1–17 (1978).
55 Hsu, H.K.; Peng, M.-T.: Hypothalamic neuron number of old female rats. Gerontology *124:* 434–440 (1978).
56 Peng, M.T.; Hsu, H.K.: No neuron loss from hypothalamic nuclei of male rats in old age. Gerontology *28:* 19–22 (1982).
57 Bellamy, D.: Cell death and the loss of structural units of organs; in Bittles, Collins, The biology of human aging: Society for the Study of Human Biology Symposium 25, pp. 119–132 (Cambridge University Press, New York 1986).

Dr. Paul Segall, Department of Physiology-Anatomy, University of California, Berkeley, CA 94720 (USA)

Interdiscipl. Topics Geront., vol. 24, pp. 21–36 (Karger, Basel 1988)

Hypothalamic-Pituitary Function in Aging Man

Judie Walton[a], *Arthur V. Everitt*[b]

[a]CSIRO, Prospect, Australia; [b]Department of Geriatric Medicine, University of Sydney, Repatriation General Hospital, Concord, Australia

Function of the Hypothalamic-Pituitary-Endocrine Axis

The hypothalamic-pituitary-endocrine axis plays a key role in coordinating activities important to our survival, enabling us to meet the challenges of an everchanging environment. It consists of a rather complex hierarchy of organs in which information is transmitted along the axis by means of hormones and neurotransmitters.

At the lower end of the axis, cells of the target glands produce anabolic and catabolic hormones which regulate many biochemical processes that profoundly affect tissue metabolism and health: carbohydrate, fat and protein synthesis and breakdown; gluconeogenesis, liver glycogen deposition, glycogenolysis, with corresponding changes in blood glucose, water, sodium and potassium renal reabsorption and excretion; germ cell maturation, somatic cell division, cell metabolism; modulation of muscle tone and excitation; effects on inflammatory, allergic and immune responses. Because of its far-reaching influences, experimental perturbations of the hypothalamic-pituitary-endocrine axis can accelerate or retard the timing with which age changes occur in various tissues of laboratory animals [1]. However, similar experiments have not been performed on humans.

Anatomy and Physiology of Neuroendocrine Interrelationships

Neurons in the hypophysiotropic area of the hypothalamus synthesize peptide hormones which regulate secretory activity in the anterior pituitary (fig. 1). After release from specific nerve endings in the median eminence of the hypothalamus, these peptide neurohormones enter the hypo-

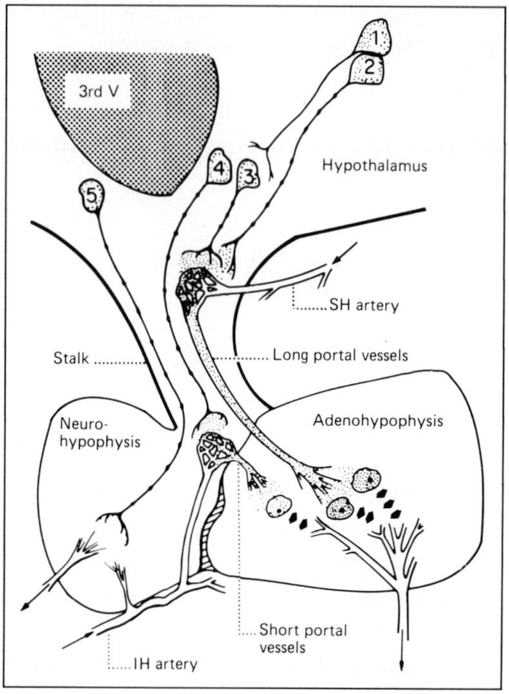

Fig. 1. Stimulation of anterior pituitary (adenohypophysis) hormone secretion (arrows) by hypothalamic neurons (1–4) mediated by releasing hormones liberated by neurons 2–4. Neuron 5 directly stimulates secretion of hormones from the posterior pituitary (neurohypophysis) [from ref. 77, with permission]. SH = Superior hypophyseal (artery), IH = inferior hypophyseal (artery). Adapted from Gay, V.L.: The hypothalamus: physiology and clinical use of releasing factors. Fert. Steril. *23:* 50 (1972). Reproduced with permission of the publisher, The American Fertility Society.

physeal portal vessels and then pass directly into the anterior pituitary where they stimulate or inhibit the release of pituitary hormones. Extrahypothalamic structures of the limbic system and the pineal body [2] also modulate pituitary function.

The anterior pituitary synthesizes at least six hormones which bear the suffix '-tropin' to indicate their attraction to a particular target gland. For each of them there is a corresponding releasing hormone (liberin). For example, thyrotropin-releasing hormone or thyroliberin, produced primarily in the hypothalamus but also within other neural and nonneural tissues, causes release of thyrotropin or thyroid-stimulating hormone

(TSH) from the pituitary. The hypothalamus also produces statins which inhibit the release of certain pituitary hormones.

Anterior pituitary hormones regulate growth, reproduction, and metabolism either directly or by stimulating function of the pituitary's target glands: the ovary, testis, adrenal cortex, thyroid, and also the liver. These endocrine glands secrete hormones which bind to cytoplasmic and membrane receptors of a wide variety of cell types throughout the body. Hypothalamic cells also have receptors responsive to gonadal, thyroid and adrenocortical hormones, thus providing feedback mechanisms for controlling their levels in the circulation.

The posterior pituitary, or neurohypophysis, is a neural extension of the hypothalamus. It stores oxytocin (OT) and vasopressin (VP) which are produced in the supraoptic and paraventricular nuclei of the hypothalamus. VP and OT neurons project from these nuclei to the neurohypophysis where the hormones are eventually released into the bloodstream (fig. 1). Fibers from VP and OT neurons innervate a large number of brain areas where the two peptides probably act as neurotransmitters [3]. Relatively high concentrations of VP and OT in the ovary suggest that they may also be locally produced there [4].

In females, OT functions in the control of lactation and labor. VP's best-understood roles are to concentrate the urine by stimulating resorption of water independently of solutes in the distal tubules and collecting ducts of kidney and also to influence blood pressure through baroreceptors.

Structure and Function of the Aging Neuroendocrine System

Structural age change is visible in at least some cell types of every organ within the hypothalamic-pituitary-endocrine axis. In general, endocrine tissues, like most other tissues, show to varying extents, an age-related tendency for cell loss and fibrosis.

Many aged tissues have reduced numbers of hormone receptors, which presumably decreases their sensitivity to circulating hormones. Even the hypothalamus and pituitary show diminished sensitivity to some hormonal feedback controls but the binding affinity of hormones to receptors on or in cells does not seem to be a component of this sensitivity loss.

Receptors in various species covering a wide range of life spans are lost from steroid responsive tissues on a comparable timescale [5]. Gregerman [6], however, makes the point that the number of receptors on a cell's surface is not fixed but varies rapidly with hormone concentration in its milieu. The ability of cells to regulate receptor number through synthesis or redistribution may vary with age although to date only a few observations are available [7]. Thus, it is not clear whether the smaller numbers of receptors in older tissues is due to decrease in receptor synthesis by aged cells or to a falloff in the total numbers of hormone-responsive cells.

Level 1: Changes in the Aging Brain (Extrahypothalamic Regions)

Within the brain, the limbic system is the main complex which communicates by means of neurotransmitters with the hypothalamic-pituitary axis. Because all hypothalamic functions, including the secretion of releasing factors for pituitary hormones, are dependent on neurotransmitter activity, it has been proposed that age-related changes in catecholamine transmitter levels may trigger a cascade of aging changes which become amplified as the effects pass down the neuroendocrine axis [8].

Neuron loss increases as a function of age in some brain structures involved in neuroendocrine control mechanisms. For example, between ages 20 and 90, the human cerebral cortex loses 30% of its cell population [9] and cells are also lost from the locus ceruleus [10]. And, in the hippocampus where pyramidal cells appear to be especially affected by the aging process [11], it has been suggested that neuron loss may influence some of the rhythmic neuroendocrine secretory processes [12].

Nevertheless, most studies measuring content of the various neurotransmitters in human autopsy tissue fail to reach a consensus and there is much disagreement in the literature whether most transmitters in specified regions of human brain increase, decrease, or show no change.

Lesioning studies in rats suggest that massive deafferentation is necessary to affect brain function so one may wonder whether age-related neuron loss is substantial enough to cause neuroendocrine dysfunction. It is important to bear in mind, though, that neuron loss is additive to structural and functional changes which develop over the decades in the surviving neuronal population, including decreases in the density of their synapses and dendritic networks 13].

Level 2: Changes in the Aging Hypothalamus

The hypothalamus is comprised of 32 pairs of nuclei which activate, control, and integrate peripheral autonomic mechanisms, endocrine activity, and many somatic functions such as water balance, body temperature, sleep, food intake, and development of secondary sex characteristics. It receives nervous input from both the periphery and higher centers, and it also receives chemical input from metabolites and hormones.

In old age, the hypothalamus appears to lose sensitivity to a variety of stimuli. The data of Dilman et al. [14] suggest that, with time, the human hypothalamus becomes less sensitive to glucose. Everitt and Huang [15] have suggested that a loss of receptors from aged hypothalamic cells may account for their reduced responsiveness.

Information about structural age change in the human hypothalamus is scant and in need of increased attention. Neurons of the supraoptic and paraventricular nuclei are markedly enlarged from 8 to 10 times their size in young individuals [16] but there is little or no evidence that they accumulate lipofuscin with time [17] or that they diminish in number. Multinucleated cells with hyperchromasia are also seen in some nuclei [16] and Blumenthal [18] has speculated that these structural differences may be due to age-related change in hormone feedback mechanisms.

Hypothalamic gonadotropin-releasing hormone stimulates the release of luteinizing hormone (LH) and follicle-stimulating hormone (FSH) from the pituitary. Gonadotropin-releasing-hormone levels are increased in the plasma of postmenopausal women [19] but to date this is the only hypothalamic hormone for which evidence of age change is documented. For example, increasing age has little effect on the interaction of growth-hormone-releasing hormone and the ability of pituitary somatotropes to respond by secreting growth hormone (GH) [20].

A characteristic of hypothalamic aging is that set points tend to change for its centers which govern physiological regulatory functions. One example of altered set point in the aged has been suggested for estrogen control of the negative feedback loop in the hypothalamus. This is based on the observation that physiologically adequate amounts of replacement estrogen are not sufficient to return postmenopausal gonadotropins to premenopausal levels [6]. Older men also have a greater steroid dose requirement for inhibition of gonadotropin secretion [21].

The hypothalamic set points which regulate VP secretion are affected by aging because in the elderly both osmoreceptor and baroreceptor responses to stimulation are subnormal [22, 23]. Some evidence also indicates altered rhythms of VP release and electrolyte secretion during aging. Whereas young people excrete twice as much urine during the day as at night, the elderly excrete nearly the same volume [24].

Level 3: Changes in the Aging Pituitary

The anterior pituitary reaches its maximum size in middle age and then gradually becomes atrophic and fibrotic in old age. It shows a loss of acidophils and in postmenopausal females gonadotropin cells are vacuolated [25]. Hyperplastic areas and small adenomas are often found, particularly prolactinomas which are common in old individuals [26].

A range of pharmacological tests has been designed to provoke hormone release from the pituitary. Despite the progressive decrease in pituitary weight with age, these tests for dynamic function have not revealed any significant impairment of pituitary tropic hormone reserve with age.

Prolactin. After menopause, plasma levels of prolactin decrease, in parallel with estrogen, to about 40% of premenopausal values. After age 64, plasma prolactin steadily increases almost to values found in young women [27]. This increase could come from the growth of pituitary prolactinomas and it was suggested [28] that prolactin might be involved in the promotion of breast cancers. In men, no change in plasma prolactin concentration has been found [28].

Gonadotropins. Serum gonadotropins, that is FSH and LH, increase in both sexes. These increases are apparently secondary reponses to a primary reduction in gonadal hormones and a resultant decrease in sex steroid feedback inhibition of the hypothalamic-pituitary axis.

In postmenopausal women, urinary FSH increases as much as 15-fold [29] and LH rises 5-fold over premenopausal levels [30], the rise eventually decreasing in very old women. Gonadotropin concentrations also correlate positively with age in men, with FSH increasing 3-fold and LH about 2-fold after age 50 [31, 32]. Baker et al. [33] suggested that the greater increase in FSH than LH in males may represent the independent regulation of FSH secretion by a seminiferous tubular factor (inhibin) which becomes deficient as tubular function decreases with age. Some of the excess LH may be biologically inactive due to impairment of pituitary enzymes responsible for glycosylation even though immunologically the LH may appear normal [34, 35].

Thyrotropin or TSH. Some authors maintain that there is no clear-cut evidence that serum TSH levels change with age [36] whereas others report that TSH increases (to more than 10 μU/ml) in elderly people [37] or a significant lowering of nighttime levels of TSH occurs in elderly subjects when compared to levels in young adults [38]. The pituitary thyrotropes may become somewhat less responsive to hypothalamic thyrotropin-releasing hormone because exogenous doses produced a smaller rise in plasma TSH in elderly subjects than in young individuals [39].

Adrenocorticotropin. Measurements of plasma adrenocorticotropin (ACTH) in 25 young and 28 elderly humans reveals no significant differences [40] and older people undergoing major surgery do not show conspicuous change in ACTH response. Also, stimulation of ACTH and β-endorphin by exogenous corticotropin-releasing factor does not change with age [41]. Moreover, the episodic secretion of ACTH which occurs at the end of normal sleep (6.00–8.00 a.m.) shows no detectable decrement in older subjects [40].

Growth Hormone. GH and the somatomedins are not only stimulatory to the development of bone and other tissues in growing animals but are also important to the maintenance of muscle mass [42], cartilage and bone [43] after growth ceases.

Loss of acidophils (which include GH-secreting cells) is a feature of pituitary involution. Old men and women show a depressed GH secretory response to stress, surgical trauma, exercise, and arginine treatment [40, 44, 45]. Plasma levels of somatomedin-C which is synthesized in the liver under GH control were lower in older than in younger subjects [46, 47]. In people aged 55 and older, the fraction of GH secreted in pulses over a 24-hour period was 29% in comparison with 81% in a younger group (18–33 years old) [46]. The 24-hour secretion of GH decreases in postmenopausal women in proportion to the fall in estradiol [46].

Level 4: Changes in the Aging Thyroid

The thyroid hormones – thyroxine (T_4) and its more potent, deiodinated metabolite triiodothyronine (T_3) – mainly function to increase the rate of cell metabolism. Although T_4 and T_3 levels in blood fall no more than by 10% between the ages of 20 and 80 [39], there is a 50% decline in T_4 production and in its uptake and degradation by target cells [48]. The basal metabolic rate falls by approximately 16% between the ages of 30 and 90 [49] but to some extent this is attributable to increase between these ages in the fat: muscle composition of the human body [50].

Most thyroids of older individuals show some degree of follicular atrophy with a small loss in weight, diminished mitoses, and fibrosis [51]. The thyroid has a lowered uptake of radioactive iodine in old age [52] and the decreased mass of metabolically active tissue could contribute to the age-related falloff in thyroid activity.

Many aging phenomena resemble aspects of hypothyroidism. In addition to lowered thyroid function and a slower metabolic rate, old people usually are cold-intolerant and they tend to have dry skin, diminished motor activity, sparseness of hair, atherosclerosis and hypercholesterolemia [53]. Slowing of the rate of T_4 disposal seems to be a feature of aging in many tissues and Gregerman [6] has suggested that it could result from decreased activity of enzymes in tissues which deiodinate or otherwise inactivate T_4. Nevertheless when stressed, as by infection, the elderly can respond with accelerated thyroid hormone metabolism [54].

Clinicians usually attribute low thyroid function to diminished output of thyroid hormones. If the hypothyroid-like condition which accompanies aging should primarily be one of depressed hormone uptake and utilization by peripheral tissues, it probably would not respond to treatment with oral T_4, unless the rise in plasma thyroid concentration is able to boost receptor numbers in aged tissues.

Changes in the Aging Ovary. Human females are born with approximately two million oocytes, most of which are subsequently destroyed by atresia [55]. During the reproductive years, oocytes mature in follicles of estrogen-secreting cells. Each month one or two mature oocytes are released into the oviduct but many more of them begin to grow and then degenerate. By the time women are about 50 years of age, their oocyte supply is virtually exhausted [56], and menstrual cycling ends. Follicle cells fail to divide and secrete estrogen, corpora lutea no longer form and produce progesterone, and plasma levels of ovarian hormones fall. The adrenal cortex partially compensates for this falloff because after menopause a substantial proportion of its androgens are converted to estrogens.

The hypothalamic-pituitary axis responds to the falloff in the production of estrogens by raising FSH and LH levels but, despite this, the ovary fails to reinstate estrogen production. Soon thereafter the female reproductive system undergoes general involution. In postmenopausal women not receiving estrogen replacement therapy, blood vessels and epithelial components of the secondary sex organs atrophy [57] and osteoporotic change tends to occur in bone. Estrogen lack is the most marked hormone deficiency in old age and failure of the ovary to respond to the high, postmenopausal levels of pituitary gonadotropins indicates that the primary age change lies in the ovary itself [15].

Changes in the Aging Testis. Unlike the ovary, the testis does not undergo an abrupt cessation of function in later life and changes take place much more gradually. Testosterone is produced by Leydig cells located in the interstitial spaces between testis tubules. The average number of Leydig cells was decreased by 44% in a 50- to 76-year-old group of men compared with another group aged 20–48 years [31]. Daily sperm production was more than 50% lower in the older men, negatively correlating with age. Age-related studies on the reserve capacity of the Leydig cells to respond to human chorionic gonadotropin have shown that both baseline and peak testosterone levels were lower in older men [32]; these results would reflect the reduced complement of normally responsive Leydig cells.

Tissue-available testosterone, including circulating free testosterone and albumin-bound testosterone, begins to decrease in middle-aged men [58] and this may not be entirely due to the smaller numbers of testosterone-producing cells. Some of the testosterone is bound to a plasma sex-hormone-binding globulin (SHBG) which increases with age, thus reducing the amount available to other tissues. Some workers have hypothesized that the increase in SHBG might be secondary to an increase in plasma estrogenic steroids since it is known that estrogens promote synthesis of SHBG by the liver. Whether estrogens do or do not increase in older men, however, is still controversial [59].

There has been conflicting data presented as to whether plasma levels of total testosterone diminish, or increase, or show no change with age. This may be related to its pattern of secretion. In young men, plasma testosterone levels fluctuate with a circadian rhythm, reaching maximum values at about 8.00 a.m. When measurements are taken in the morning testosterone values in old subjects are substantially lower than in young ones [60]. However, this rhythmic pattern is apparently lost in older men so when testosterone values of the two groups are measured in the afternoon, well after the peak, plasma levels tend to be similar.

In old age, testosterone deficit leads to involution of male accessory sex glands. The prostate and seminal vesicles atrophy and seminal fluid is reduced in volume and viscosity [61]. Spermatogenesis may be normal even in extreme old age but generalized hypospermatogenesis is common [62].

Changes in the Aging Adrenal Cortex. The adrenal cortex synthesizes glucocorticoids and androgens in response to ACTH, and aldosterone in response to angiotensin II and ACTH.

In aging men and women, the adrenal gland decreases in weight and cortical nodules are frequently seen. The senescent cortex tends to undergo fibrotic change with decreases in epithelial cell number and in steroid-containing lipid. Vascular dilatation and hemorrhage are common [63].

Cells of the zona reticularis accumulate lipofuscin [64], a marker of cellular aging. Synthesis of the main sex hormone, dehydroepiandrosterone falls off steadily after the 3rd decade [65], decreasing by age 60 to approximately one third of the amount secreted at age 30. In postmenopausal women, there is at least a 50% increased conversion of dehydroepiandrosterone to estrone which can to some extent compensate for the decline with age in gonadal hormone production [66].

Aldosterone secretion [67] and levels of plasma aldosterone and renin activity show a large reduction in healthy normotensive subjects above age 60 when compared with young adults [68]. This leads to decreased activity of the renin-angiotensin-aldosterone system in the elderly [69].

Rates of cortisol synthesis have not been directly determined for humans of different ages. Plasma cortisol levels remain constant with age but the early morning peak secretion occurs a few hours later in older subjects [70]. As estrogen stimulates the synthesis in liver of corticosteroid binding protein [71], postmenopausal women could have a greater percentage of their plasma cortisol in the unbound form.

There is evidence that tissues in the aged body utilize glucocorticoids to a lesser extent [72]. Cortisol removal from circulating blood is much slower in old age [73] and some organs in older subjects have fewer corticosteroid receptors. For example, a group of people aged 66–80 years were found to have 70% less glucocorticoid binding per unit wet weight in livers than a group of 30- to 40-year olds [74]. This occurs without change in the concentration of circulating cortisol levels so it implies an inability of aged human cells to produce receptors and/or reflects substantial cell loss.

Interactions Which Affect Aging along the Hypothalamic-Pituitary Axis

Neuroendocrine interrelationships are complex and as the hypothalamic-pituitary endocrine axis utilizes feedback to function as a loop, it is often difficult to pinpoint the locus of an age-related change. It is possible for a small decline in secretion of a target gland hormone (e.g. cortisol) to be compensated for by an increased secretion of the appropriate pituitary tropin (e.g. ACTH) without change in the plasma level of either hormone. Detection of small age changes in plasma levels may require a study of hormone pulses over 24 h.

Age changes have been demonstrated at all levels of the hypothalamic-pituitary axis as well as in other tissues which affect the function of this system. Rates of hormone synthesis and utilization are more meaningful than plasma concentrations which in many cases are maintained by feedback at relatively constant values throughout life. Lower tissue utilization of a hormone, such as T_4 or cortisol, leads to a homeostatic slowing of its synthesis. Conversely, if a hormone is synthesized at a lowered rate, that may also affect its rates of uptake and utilization. Hence, absence of difference in plasma levels of a particular hormone in young and old subjects should not be interpreted to mean that the organ which secretes it shows no age change [6].

Reduced tissue responsiveness to a hormone in old age may be due to loss of receptors and to the loss of cells. The synthesis of hormone receptors may diminish with time in each cell of an aging cohort, making the tissue generally less responsive to hormones. However, atrophy-related cell loss could also contribute to decrease in tissue receptor numbers in a way that would affect hormone uptake and removal from the circulation. Because the pituitary, gonads, adrenal cortex and thyroid gland all show some degree of atrophy with time, they have fewer cells available to respond to hormones from higher levels and to produce their own hormones.

Apart from the hypothalamic-pituitary-endocrine axis, other organ systems intimately affect all other body tissues, particularly the vasculature and the nervous system. As organ systems cannot be functionally dissociated from each other, age damage to one can also produce change in the others. For example, the age-related decrease in vascularity of the anterior pituitary [75] may impair delivery of oxygen and hypothalamic hormones as well as removal of its own hormones and waste products. Conversely, the postmenopausal falloff in estrogen level is probably deleterious to the cardiovascular system since estrogen replacement therapy reduces the incidence of coronary artery disease, atherosclerosis, and congestive heart failure [76].

Age-related malfunction in the brain causes decline and disappearance of circadian pulses in the secretion of most hormones. However, to date, there is no other clear evidence that a small change in brain function generates a cascade of deleterious effects which are amplified as they pass down the axis, as proposed by Finch [8] for the rodent.

In conclusion, the hypothalamus and pituitary have reserve capacities for normal production of most hormones throughout adult life. But, in later years, glands situated lower on the neuroendocrine axis (thyroid, adrenal cortex, gonads) exhibit diminishing rates of secretion and their hormones are utilized at progressively lower rates.

References

1 Everitt, A.V.: The hypothalamic-pituitary control of aging and age-related pathology. Exp. Gerontol. *8:* 265–277 (1973).

2 Romijn, H.T.: The pineal, a tranquilizing organ? Life Sci. *23:* 2257–2274 (1978).

3 Buijs, R.M.: The ultrastructural localization of amines, amino acids and peptides in the brain; in Buijs, Pevet, Swaab, Chemical transmission in the brain. The role of amines, amino acids and peptides. Progress in brain research, vol. 55, pp. 167–183 (Elsevier, Amsterdam 1982).

4 Wathes, D.C.; Pickering, B.T.; Swann, R.W.; Porter, D.G.: Neurohypophysial hormones in the human ovary. Lancet *ii:* 410–412 (1982).

5 Roth, G.S.: Age-related changes in specific glucocorticoid binding by steroid responsive tissues of rats. Endocrinology *94:* 82–90 (1974).

6 Gregerman, R.I.: Mechanisms of age-related alterations of hormone secretion and action. An overview of 30 years of progress. Exp. Gerontol. *21:* 345–365 (1986).

7 Dax, E.M.: Receptors and associated membrane events in aging. Rev. Biol. Res. Aging *2:* 315–366 (1985).

8 Finch, C.E.: The regulation of physiological changes during mammalian aging. Q. Rev. Biol. *51:* 49–83 (1976).

9 Brody, H.: Organization of the cerebral cortex. II. A study of aging in the human cerebral cortex. J comp. Neurol. *102:* 511–556 (1955).

10 Vijayashankar, N.; Brody, H.J.: A quantitative study of the pigmented neurons in the nuclei locus coeruleus and subcoeruleus in man as related to aging. Neuropath. exp. Neurol. *38:* 490–497 (1979).

11 Ball, M.J.: Neuronal loss, neurofibrillary tangles and granulovacuolar degeneration in the hippocampus with ageing and dementia. A quantitative study. Acta neuropath. *37:* 111–118 (1977).

12 Clemens, J.A.: Morphological changes in the hypothalamus and other brain areas influencing endocrine function during aging; in Meites, Neuroendocrinology of aging, pp. 31–39 (Plenum, New York 1983).

13 Peters, A.; Vaughan, D.W.: Central nervous system; in Johnson, Aging and cell structure, vol. 1, pp. 1–34 (Plenum Press, New York 1981).

14 Dilman, V.M.; Bobrov, J.F.; Ostroumova, M.N.; Lvovich, E.G.; Vishnevsky, A.S.; Anisimov, V.N.; Vasiljeva, I.A.: Hypothalmic mechanisms of ageing and of specific age pathology. III. Sensitivity threshold of hypothalamo-pituitary complex to homeostatic stimuli in energy systems. Exp. Gerontol. *14:* 217–224 (1979).

15 Everitt, A.V.; Huang, C.Y.: The hypothalamus, neuroendocrine and autonomic nervous systems in aging; in Birren, Sloane, Handbook on mental health in aging, pp. 100–132 (Prentice Hall, Englewood Cliffs 1980).
16 Von Buttlar-Brentano, K.: Zur Lebensgeschichte des Nuclear basilis, tubermammalaris, supraopticus und paraventriculus unter normalen und pathogenen Bedingungen. J. Hirnforsch. *1:* 337–419 (1954).
17 Azcoaga, J.E.: Senilidad de las neuronas de los nucleos magnocelulares del hipotalamo. Arch. Histol. *9:* 40–48 (1965).
18 Blumenthal, H.T.: Immunological aspects of the aging brain; in Terry, Gershon, Aging. Neurobiology of aging. vol. 3, pp. 313–334 (Raven Press, New York 1976).
19 Seyler, L.E., Jr.; Reichlin, S.: Luteinizing hormone-releasing factor (LRF) in plasma of post-menopausal women. J. clin. Endocr. Metab. *37:* 197–203 (1973).
20 Pavlov, E.P.; Harman, S.M.; Merriam, G.R.; Gelato, M.C.; Blackman, M.R.: Responses of growth hormone (GH) and somatomedin-C to GH-releasing hormone in healthy aging men. J. clin. Endocr. Metab. *62:* 595–600 (1986).
21 Muta, K.; Kato, K.; Akamine, Y.; Ibayashi, H.: Age-related changes in the feedback regulation of gonadotropin secretion by sex steroids in men. Acta endocr., Copenh. *96:* 154–162 (1981).
22 Mukherjee, A.P.; Coni, N.K.; Davison, W.: Osmoreceptor function among the elderly. Geront. clin. *15:* 227–233 (1973).
23 Rowe, J.W.; Minaker, K.L.; Sparrow, D.; Robertson, G.L.: Age-related failure of volume-pressure-mediated vasopressin release. J. clin. Endocr. Metab. *54:* 661–664 (1982).
24 Kirkland, J.L.; Lye, M.; Levy, D.W.; Banerjee, A.K.: Patterns of urine flow and electrolyte secretion in healthy elderly people. Br. med. J. *287:* 1665–1667 (1983).
25 Severinghaus, A.E.: Cytology of the anterior pituitary of the postmenopausal woman. J. clin. Endocrinol. *4:* 583–588 (1944).
26 Kovacs, K.; Horvath, E.; Corenblum, B.; Sirek, A.M.T.; Penz, G.; Ezrin, C.: Pituitary chromophobe adenomas consisting of prolactin cells. A histologic, immunocytological and electron microscopic study. Virchows Arch Abt. A Path. Anat. Histol., *366:* 113–123 (1975).
27 Bulbrook, R.D.; Wang, D.Y.; Hayward, J.L.; Kwa, H.G.; Cleton, F.: Plasma prolactin levels and age in a female population: relation to breast cancer. Int. J. Cancer *28:* 43–45 (1981).
28 Blackman, M.R.; Kowatch, M.A.; Wehmann, R.E.; Harman, S.M.: Basal serum prolactin levels and prolactin responses to constant infusion of thyrotropin releasing hormone in healthy aging men. J. Geront. *41:* 699–705 (1986).
29 Coble, Y.D., Jr.; Kohler, P.O.; Cargille, C.M.; Ross, G.T.: Production rates and metabolic clearance rates of human follicle-stimulating hormone in premenopausal and postmenopausal women. J. clin. Invest. *48:* 359–363 (1969).
30 Kohler, P.O.; Ross, G.T.; Odell, W.D.: Metabolic clearance and production rates of human luteinizing hormone in pre- and postmenopausal women. J. clin. Invest. *47:* 38–47 (1968).
31 Neaves, W.B.; Johnson, L.; Porter, J.C.; Parker, L.R., Jr.; Petty, C.S.: Leydig cell numbers, daily sperm production and serum gonadotropin levels in aging men. J. clin. Endocr. Metab. *59:* 756–763 (1984).

32 Mazzi, C.; Riva, L.R.; Bernasconi, D.: Gonadotropins and plasma testosterone in senescence; in James, Serio, Martini, The endocrine function of human testis, vol. 2, pp. 51–62 (Academic Press, New York 1974).
33 Baker, H.W.G.; Bremner, W.J.; Burger, H.S.; Kretser, D.M. de; Dulmanis, A.; Eddie, L.W.; Hudson, B.; Keogh, E.J.; Lee, V.W.K.; Rennie, G.C.: Testicular control of follicle-stimulating hormone secretion. Recent Prog. Horm. Res. *32:* 429–476 (1976).
34 Marrama, P.; Montanini, V.; Celani, M.F.; Carani, C.; Cioni, K.; Bazzani, M.; Cavani, D.; Baraghini, G.F.: Decrease in luteinizing hormone biological activity/immunoreactivity ratio in elderly men. Maturitas *5:* 223–231 (1984).
35 Warner, B.A.; Dufau, M.L.; Santen, R.J.: Effects of aging and illness on the pituitary testicular axis in men: qualitative as well as quantitative changes in luteinizing hormone. J. clin. Endocr. Metab. *60:* 263–268 (1985).
36 Wagner, H.; Hengst, K.; Hossdorf, T.: The aged thyroid gland; in Platt, Geriatrics, Part II pp. 102–142 (Springer, Berlin 1983).
37 Sawin, C.T.; Castelli, W.P.; Hershman, J.M.; McNamara, P.; Bacharach, P.: The aging thyroid: thyroid deficiency in the Framington study. Archs intern Med. *145:* 1386–1388 (1985).
38 Barreca, T.; Franceschini, R.; Messina, V.; Botarro, L.; Rolandi, E.: 24-hour thyroid-stimulating hormone secretory pattern in elderly men. Gerontology *31:* 119–123 (1985).
39 Harman, S.M.; Wehmann, R.E.; Blackman, M.R.: Pituitary-thyroid hormone economy in healthy aging men: basal indices of thyroid function and thyrotropin responses to constant infusions of thyrotropin releasing hormone. J. clin. Endocr. Metab. *58:* 320–331 (1984).
40 Blichert-Toft, M.: Secretion of corticotrophin and somatotrophin by the senescent adenohypophysis in man. Acta endocr. *78:* suppl. 195, pp. 15–154 (1975).
41 Chiarini, V.; Graziano, E.; Cremonini, N.; Leandri, P.; Zampa, G.A.: Human corticotropin-releasing factor (h-CRF) test in the aging; in Vezzadini, Facchini, Labo, Neuroendocrine system and aging, pp. 133–137 (Eurage, Rijswijk 1986).
42 Rudman, D.: Growth hormone, body composition, and aging. J. Am. Geriat. Soc. *33:* 800–807 (1985).
43 Canalis, E.: The hormonal and local regulation of bone formation. Endocr. Rev. *4:* 62–77 (1983).
44 Dudl, R.J.; Ensinck, J.W.; Palmer, H.E.; Williams, R.H.: Effect of age on growth hormone secretion in man. J. clin. Endocr. Metab. *37:* 11–16 (1973).
45 Bazzare, T.L.; Johanson, A.J.; Huseman, C.A.; Varma, M.M.; Blizzard, R.M.: Human growth hormone changes with age, in Pecile, Muller, Growth hormone and related peptides, pp. 261–270 (Excerpta Medica, Amsterdam 1976).
46 Ho, K.Y.; Evans, W.S.; Blizzard, R.M.; Veldhuis, J.D.; Merriam, G.R.; Samojlik, E.; Furlanetto, R.; Rogol, A.D.; Kaiser, D.L.; Thorner, M.O.: Effects of sex and age on the 24-hour profile of growth hormone secretion in man: importance of endogenous estradiol concentrations. J. clin. Endocr. Metab. *64:* 51–58 (1987).
47 Florini, J.R.; Prinz, P.N.; Vitiello, M.V.; Hintz, R.L.: Somatomedin-C levels in healthy young and old men: relationship to peak and 24-hour integrated levels of growth hormone. J. Geront. *40:* 2–7 (1985).
48 Gregerman, R.I.; Gaffney, G.W.; Shock, N.W.: Thyroxine turnover in euthyroid

man with special reference to changes with age. J. clin. Invest. *41.* 2065–2074 (1962).
49 Shock, N.W.; Yiengst, M.J.: Age changes in basal respiratory measurements and metabolism in males. J. Geront. *10:* 31–40 (1955).
50 Tzankoff, S.P.; Norris, A.H.: Effect of muscle mass decrease on age-related BMR changes. J. appl. Physiol. *43:* 4001–1006 (1977).
51 Andrew, W.: The anatomy of aging in man and animals (Grune & Stratton, New York 1971).
52 Oddie, T.H.; Myhill, J.; Pirnique, F.G.; Fisher, D.A.: Effect of age and sex on the radioiodine uptake in euthyroid subjects. J. clin. Endocrinol. *28:* 776–782 (1968).
53 Korenchevsky, V.: Physiological and pathological ageing (Karger, Basel 1961).
54 Gregerman, R.I.; Solomon, N.: Acceleration of thyroxine and triiodothyronine turnover during bacterial pulmonary infections and fever: implications for the functional state of the thyroid during stress and in senescence. J. clin. Endocr. Metab. *27:* 93–105 (1967).
55 Baker, T.G.: A quantitative and cytological study of germ cells in human ovaries. Proc. R. Soc. Ser. B. *158:* 417–433 (1963).
56 Eckstein, P.: Endocrine activities of the ovary; in Zucker, Weir, The ovary, vol. 2, pp. 275–313 (Academic Press, New York 1977).
57 Timiras, P.S.; Meisami, E.: Changes in gonadal function; in Timiras, Developmental physiology and aging, pp. 527–541 (Macmillan, New York 1972).
58 Nankin, H.R.; Calkins, J.H.: Decreased bioavailable testosterone in aging normal and impotent men. J. clin. Endocr. Metab. *63:* 1418–1420 (1986).
59 Harman, S.M.: Relation of the neuroendocrine system to reproductive decline in men; in Meites, Neuroendocrinology of aging, pp. 203–220 (Plenum Press, New York 1983).
60 Bremner, W.J.; Vitiello, M.V.; Prinz, P.N.: Loss of circadian rhythmicity in blood testosterone levels with aging in normal men. J. clin. Endocr. Metab. *56:* 1278–1281 (1983).
61 Steward, V.W.; Brandes, D.: The accessory male sex glands and their changes with age; in Bourne, Structural aspects of aging, pp. 399–414 (Hafner, New York 1961).
62 Baker, H.W.G.; Burger, H.G.; Kretser, D.M. de; Hudson, B.: Endocrinology of aging: pituitary-testicular axis; in James, Endocrinology, vol. 2, pp. 479–483 (Excerpta Medica, Amsterdam 1977).
63 Gregerman, R.I.; Bierman, E.L.: Aging and hormones; in Williams, Textbook of endocrinology; 6th ed., pp. 1193–1212 (Saunders, Philadelphia 1981).
64 Planel, H.; Guilhelm, A.: Contribution à l'étude histochimique des pigments de la glande surrénale du cobaye en fonction de l'âge. C.R. Soc. Biol. (Paris) *149:* 1504–1507 (1955).
65 De Peretti, E.; Forest, M.G.: Pattern of plasma dehydroepiandrosterone sulfate levels in humans from birth to adulthood: evidence for testicular production. J. clin. Endocr. Metab. *47:* 572–577 (1978).
66 Studd, J.W.W.; Thom, M.H.: Ovarian failure and ageing. Clin. Endocrinol. Metab. *10:* 89–113 (1981).
67 Hegstad, R.; Brown, R.D.; Jiang, N.-S.; Kao, P.; Weinshilboum, R.M.; Strong, C.; Wisgerhof, M.: Aging and aldosterone. Am. J. Med. *74:* 442–448 (1983).

68 Noth, R.H.; Lassman, N.; Tan, S.Y.; Fernandez-Cruz, A.; Mulrow, P.J.: Age and the renin-aldosterone system. Archs. intern. Med. *137:* 1414–1417 (1977).
69 Sambhi, M.P.; Crane, M.G.; Genest, J.: Essential hypertension: newer concepts about mechanisms. Ann. intern. Med. *79:* 411–424 (1973).
70 Sherman, B.; Wysham, C.; Pfohl, B.: Age-related changes in the circadian rhythm of plasma cortisol in man. J. clin. Endocr. Metab. *61:* 439:443 (1985).
71 Larsson-Cohn, U.: Some biochemical consequences of postmenopausal hormonal replacement treatment; in Van Keep, Utian, Vermeulen, The controversial climacteric, pp. 29–37 (MTP Press, Lancaster 1982).
72 Minaker, K.L.; Meneilly, G.S.; Rowe, J.W.: Endocrine systems; in Finch, Schneider, Handbook of the biology of aging; 2nd ed., pp. 433–456 (Van Nostrand & Reinhold, New York 1985).
73 Samuels, L.T.: Effects of aging on steroid metabolism; in Engel, Pincus, Hormones and the aging process, pp. 21–38 (Academic Press, New York 1956).
74 Singer, S.; Ito, H.; Litwack, G.: ^{3}H-cortisol binding by young and old human liver cytosol proteins in vitro. Int. J. Biochem. *4:* 569–573 (1973).
75 Shanklin, B.P.: Age changes in the histology of the human pituitary. Acta anat. *19:* 290–304 (1953).
76 Hammond, C.B.; Jelovsek, F.R.; Lee, K.L.; Creasman, W.T.; Parker, R.T.: Effects of long-term estrogen replacement therapy. I. Metabolic. Am. J. Obstet. Gynec. *133:* 525–536 (1979).
77 Gay, V.L.: The hypothalamus: physiology and clinical use of releasing factors. Fert. Steril. *23:* 50–63 (1972).

Dr. Judie Walton, CSIRO, PO Box 239, Blacktown, NSW 2148 (Australia)

Interdiscipl. Topics Geront., vol. 24, pp. 37–50 (Karger, Basel 1988)

Neuroendocrine Basis of Aging in the Rat

Joseph Meites[1]

Department of Physiology, Michigan State University, East Lansing, Mich., USA

Introduction

We believe the genome controls aging processes largely via the homeostatic and integrative mechanisms of the body, which means primarily the neuroendocrine, immune, and cell-to-cell communicating systems. Of these we consider the neuroendocrine system to be the most important, since it regulates to a greater or lesser degree practically every organ and tissue in the body, including the immune system. The neuroendocrine hypothesis of aging is based on the view that inasmuch as the neuroendocrine system exerts such important control of body functions during early and mature life, it must have an equally important role during the later period of life. Research on the neuroendocrinology of aging during the last 15–20 years largely supports this hypothesis. We define aging in terms of decreases in function of organs and tissues, associated with reduced ability to maintain homeostasis.

Study of the neuroendocrinology of aging in the rat is not only of interest for its own sake, but also because of the light it sheds on the general problem of aging in all species, including man. The rat is the most widely used animal for neuroendocrine investigations, and is one of the two most

[1] Work from our laboratory was aided in part by NIH grant AG00416 from the National Institute of Aging. I am indebted to Dr. Victoria Kingsbury for editorial assistance and for typing the manuscript, and to Dr. Rodolfo Goya and Kathleen Quigley for their critical review of the manuscript.

widely used animal species for aging studies; the other is the mouse. Use of the rat has many advantages: there is a considerable body of information already available on the neuroendocrinology of aging in this species; rats are available in large numbers as genetically pure or outbred strains; they can be maintained under uniform conditions of nutrition, temperature, humidity, sanitation, and handling; and they have a sufficient supply of blood to obtain many samples for radioimmunoassays of hormones. Several differences in the neuroendocrine control of aging have been uncovered in the rat as compared to man, but a number of interesting similarities have also been demonstrated. Overall, therefore, the rat has proven to be a worthy model for such studies.

We have studied the relation of the neuroendocrine system to three important aging events in the life of the rat: the decline in reproductive functions, development of numerous mammary and pituitary tumors, and the decrease in growth hormone (GH), somatomedin secretion, and protein synthesis. We have reviewed these three aging phenomena in the rat previously [1], and shall consider here their common neuroendocrine characteristics, the possible causes for the dysfunctions that develop in the neuroendocrine system with age, and the relation of some other theories of aging to neuroendocrine aging.

Common Characteristics of Neuroendocrine Aging in the Rat

Changes in Hypothalamic Function

There is now convincing evidence that dysfunctions that develop in the hypothalamus with age are primarily but not exclusively responsible for the above three aging events in the rat. For example, when the ovaries or pituitary of young rats were transplanted to old female rats after removing their own ovaries or pituitary, there was no resumption of estrous cycles; on the other hand, when the ovaries or pituitary of old noncycling rats were transplanted to young rats after removing their own ovaries or pituitary, cycling resumed in many of the young rats [2–4]. Also, when ovaries or testes were removed from old and young rats, the rise in circulating luteinizing hormone (LH) levels was significantly lower in the old than in the young rats [5]. Other evidence will be cited demonstrating that direct changes occur in hypothalamic function during aging in the rat.

The hypothalamus contains two substances that are of particular importance in regulating endocrine functions, namely hypophysiotropic releasing or release-inhibiting peptide hormones that directly control pituitary function, and neurotransmitters that modulate release of the hypothalamic hormones into the hypophysial portal vessels. The hypophysiotropic hormones originate in neurons of the hypothalamus, whereas the hypothalamic neurotransmitters originate in neurons of the hypothalamus and midbrain. There are important interconnections between the hypothalamus and other areas of the brain, and the hypothalamus receives as well as transmits information to these areas.

Relatively little is known of the changes that occur in hypophysiotropic hormone secretion during aging. Decreases have been reported with aging in hypothalamic content of gonadotropin-releasing hormone (GnRH) [6, 7] and thyrotropin-releasing hormone (TRH) [8], and these have been interpreted as indicative of reduced release of these hormones. However, it is well recognized that measurements of tissue content of hormones do not distinguish among synthesis, release, and storage. More meaningful observations were reported when hypothalamic tissue from old and young rats was incubated in vitro and subjected to perfusion with hypermolar potassium. Under these conditions, less TRH [9] and more somatostatin [10] were released by tissue from old than from young rats. Also, less growth-hormone-releasing hormone (GHRH) was released from incubated hypothalamic tissue of old than of young rats [Miki, pers. commun.]. Apparently, sufficient amounts of GnRH, TRH, and GHRH are present in the hypothalamus of old rats to induce release of their corresponding pituitary hormones, but what is lacking is sufficient stimulus to induce their release. The two catecholamines (CAs), norepinephrine (NE) and dopamine (DA), are critically deficient in the hypothalamus of old rats [11, 12]. These are important because NE is the major neurotransmitter that promotes GnRH release in the rat, DA acts directly on the pituitary to inhibit prolactin (PRL) release, and both NE and DA stimulate GH release in man as well as in the rat [1, 11–13]. These neurotransmitters may also influence somatostatin release. Reductions in NE and DA *content* and *turnover* have been reported in many areas of the hypothalamus of old rats, including decreases in the median eminence, medial basal hypothalmus, preoptic area, and anterior hypothalamus [11, 12]. A decrease in DA in hypophysial portal blood of old rats also was reported [14]. Other neurotransmitters in the hypothalamus may also be involved in the changes that occur in release of hypothalamic and pituitary hormones with age, but little is known about this at present. Serotonin content and turnover in the hypothalamus of old rats appear to undergo little or no change [11, 15], but the ratio of serotonin to NE increases as a result of the decline in NE activity. Since serotonin may be involved in the cyclic release of GnRH, the change in ratio of serotonin to NE activity may be partly responsible for failure of ovulation in old constant-estrous rats.

Changes in Functions of the Pituitary, Target Glands, and Other Hormone-Responsive Tissues

The pituitary, target glands, and the tissues they stimulate can undergo changes that alter their responsiveness to hormones. For example, we have reported that pituitary release of LH in response to administration of GnRH is significantly lower in old than in young male and female rats [16]. This was observed not to be due to a reduction in GnRH receptors in the pituitary of the old rats [17], but rather to postreceptor changes in the gonadotropic cells. There is also evidence that the gonads of old male and female rats become less responsive to gonadotropic hormone stimulation, and the uterus less responsive to estrogen stimulation [18], the latter apparently resulting from loss of estrogen receptors [19]. A decrease in estrogen receptors in the hypothalamus has also been reported [3], and may be partially responsible for the reduced ability of estrogen to elicit LH release in old rats. Under in vivo conditions, corticotropin-releasing hormone was found to be less effective in releasing adrenocorticotropic hormone and corticosterone in old than in young rats [20]. Pituitary GH release in response to GHRH administration in vivo was lower in old than in young rats, and apparently is caused by increased somatostatin release from the hypothalamus; somatostatin directly antagonizes GHRH action on the pituitary (see chapter by Sonntag and Meites). There is also evidence for an increase in GHRH receptors in the liver of old as compared to young female rats [21], which appears to be related to the decrease in circulating GH levels. An exception is the greater response of pituitary PRL cells to estrogen stimulation in aging female rats [2]. This may be partly responsible for the increase in PRL secretion in old rats.

Aging Changes First Appear Relatively Early in Life of the Rat

A third feature of the three aging events studied in the rat is that they first appear when the rats have reached only the first third to half of their maximum life span (about 3 years), and progress thereafter. Female rats already show irregular estrous cycles by 7–10 months of age, and by 10–15 months of age most have ceased to cycle and enter a constant estrous state characterized by ovaries with well-developed follicles but no ovulation; later they may enter pseudopregnant or anestrous states [1, 2]. During the constant-estrous state, PRL secretion begins to increase and a few female rats develop mammary tumors. Most of the mammary and pituitary tumors develop much later and are the result of the progressive increase in PRL secretion. Pulsatile GH secretion in female rats is already reduced by about 50% at 11 months of age when compared to GH values in female rats 4–5 months old [22]. This may be responsible for the characteristic body growth stasis seen in mature female rats [23]. Middle-aged and older rats also show a significant fall in serum levels of somatomedin [24]. The thymus, a key component of the immune system, shows a marked reduction in size and function at the time of puberty, due to the increase in gonadal hormone secretion which occurs at this time. In human subjects, declines in many body functions also begin relatively early in life. From 30 to 80 years of age a progressive decline was reported in basal metabolism, cardiac index, vital capacity, renal blood flow, nerve conduction velocity, and other body functions [25]. Therefore aging is a phenomenon that begins relatively early in life, and progresses thereafter. What is observed during later life and senescence is believed to represent an accumulation of the decrements in body functions that had their beginnings earlier in life.

Correction of Hypothalamic Deficiences Can Delay or Reverse Aging Changes

A fourth feature of the three aging changes in body functions studied in the rat is that they can all be delayed or reversed by treatments that correct the hypothalamic deficiences that develop in aging rats. Thus, administration of *L*-dopa or other drugs that increase CAs in the hypothalamus and brain generally delayed loss of estrous cycles, and reinitiated cycles in old rats that had ceased to cycle [1]. Direct electrical stimulation of the preoptic area [26] or injections of GnRH or LH induced ovulation in old constant-estrous rats. The two latter treatments show that the pituitary and ovaries of these old rats remain responsive to hormone stimulation even though their responses may be reduced. Administration of *L*-dopa or dopaminergic ergot drugs also induced regression of mammary and pituitary tumors. *L*-Dopa administration has also been shown to elevate pulsatile GH secretion in old male rats to the same levels as in young male rats, and to increase protein synthesis in diaphragm muscle; injections of GH raised protein synthesis in diaphragm muscle of old male rats to the same levels as in young rats, and significantly increased the weights of the heart, kidney, liver, spleen, and thymus (see chapter by Sonntag and Meites).

It is of interest that some of the aging events that normally occur in older rats can be produced in younger rats by reducing hypothalamic CA activity. Thus chronic administration of neuroleptic drugs or estrogen, both of which inhibit CA activity, can induce cessation of estrous cycles by decreasing GnRH and gonadotropin secretion, and elicit development of mammary tumors by promoting PRL secretion [27]. Prolonged estrogen treatment also results in development of pituitary tumors in rats and mice [28]. This further emphasizes the predominant influence of the hypothalamus in initiating these well-recognized aging events in the rat.

Possible Causes of Neuroendocrine Dysfunctions in Aging Rats

There are many possible causes for the changes in function of the neuroendocrine system during aging in the rat. The role of the genome in aging of the neuroendocrine system is unknown, and there is no evidence for the presence of specific aging genes in the body. Since changes in hypothalamic function are believed to be primarily responsible for the aging developments we have studied in the rat, we shall emphasize primarily the role of agents that may reduce its functional capactiy. Some agents that are harmful to neurons in the hypothalamus may also damage or destroy cells in other components of the neuroendocrine system (pituitary, target, glands, and target tissues).

A significant loss of neurons was reported during aging in the arcuate nucleus, medial preoptic area, and ventromedial and lateral hypothalamic nuclei [3]. These neurons are critical for secretion of neurotransmitters and hypophysiotropic hormones, and their damage or destruction may partly account for the three aging developments studied in the rat. This is indicated, for example, by the reports that transplantation of hypothalamic tissue from newborn or fetal rats into the hypothalamus of old female rats can reestablish estrous cycles (see Huang, this publication). The decline and cessation of cycling in aging female rats may also be due in part to loss of estrogen receptors by these neurons.

Damage to neurons in the arcuate nucleus and medial basal hypothalamus, similar to that seen in untreated old rats, was induced in young rats by administration of a long-acting estrogen [29]. Our laboratory observed that implantation of an estrogen capsule into young rats for 30 days specifically injured dopaminergic neurons in the arcuate nucleus [30], the source of most of the DA that inhibits PRL secretion. The arcuate nucleus also serves as an intermediate pathway between the preoptic area which regulates ovulation, and the median eminence from which GnRH is released to the pituitary. Damage to hypothalamic neurons by estrogen action probably occurs during the many recurrent estrous cycles during reproductive life, and also during the constant-estrous state. Such damage by estrogen probably accounts for the results reported when rats or mice were ovariectomized relatively early in life and implanted with ovaries many months later, with the result that estrous cycles resumed and continued for many months beyond the period when estrous cycles ceased in intact control rats [2, 31]. Presumably, the long period when the animals were free of estrogen as a result of ovariectomy extended the functions of hypothalamic neurons involved in control of estrous cycles.

Chronically elevated circulating PRL levels from a pituitary tumor transplant were reported to damage dopaminergic neurons in the arcuate nucleus and median eminence of rats, as indicated by shrinkage of the soma and distortion of dendrites [32]. Since it is well established that estrogens can increase PRL secretion, it is possible that the damage to neurons produced by estrogen is mediated in part via increased PRL secretion. Short periods of elevated PRL levels in the blood are known to increase DA activity in the hypothalamus, but persistent high levels of circulating PRL apparently can damage DA neurons.

The chronic action of other hormones may also injure neurons in the brain. Adrenal glucocorticoid hormones have been reported to damage or destroy neurons in the hippocampus [33], an area that influences hypothalamic function. A reduction in glucocorticoid receptors in the hippocampus has also been noted [19], but its relation to damage of neurons by glucocorticoids is not clear. A deficiency of testosterone induced by castration of male rats was recently found to result in a dramatic reduction in dendritic length and soma size of motoneurons in the spinal cord, which could be reversed by testosterone administration [34]. It is possible that the decrease in testosterone secretion in aging male rats results in similar damage to hypothalamic and other brain neurons. The effects of other hormones on hypothalamic neurons during prolonged periods of life also remain to be studied.

Changes in tissue concentrations and activity of enzymes involved in synthesis and metabolism of brain neurotransmitters have been reported in aging rats. There is evidence for a reduction in tyrosine hydroxylase, the rate-limiting enzyme for CA synthesis, in the hypothalamus and other brain areas [31]. The neurons containing this enzyme were observed to take up estrogen [35], which may damage these neurons and result in reduced activity. There is also some evidence in old mice for a decrease in brain dopamine β-hydroxylase [31], which converts DA to NE. Monoamine oxidase, the major enzyme that catabolizes CAs, was reported to be increased in the brain and hypothalamus during aging [36]. The causes for these changes in enzymes in the brain during aging are not clear at present.

Other agents that may injure or induce loss of hypothalamic neurons with age include 'free radicals', 'cross-linkages', and cellular debris (lipofuscin). An increase in lipofuscin has been reported in brain neurons and in cells of endocrine glands [37], but it is not clear whether this interferes with cellular functions. There is no evidence as yet that free radicals or cross-linkages injure components of the neuroendocrine system, although this remains a possibility. Whether toxins in the environment can injure neurons or other components of the neuroendocrine system is unknown at present. It is also possible that endogenous toxins are produced in the body. Neurotoxins have been developed that can specifically injure catecholaminergic neurons, e.g. 6-hydroxydopamine. Monosodium glutamate, when administered to young rats or mice, is known to specifically destroy neurons in the arcuate nucleus.

Finally, there is the question as to whether normal daily 'wear and tear' during a prolonged period of life can result in damage to components of the neuroendocrine system. Underfeeding has been demonstrated to delay aging and preserve the integrity of various organs and tissues in the body, to preserve immune functions, to inhibit tumor formation, and to prolong life in rats and other rodent species [38]. Underfeeding is known to reduce neuroendocrine function, resulting in decreases in brain CA activity [39], release of hypothalamic peptide hormones [40], and secretion of pituitary and target gland hormones [40–42]. These lead to reduced function by body organs and tissues, and decreased basal metabolism. We believe that these are the major mechanisms by which restricted food intake exerts its beneficial effects on body functions. Hypophysectomy can also delay aging changes in some body tissues, but it does not prolong life unless glucocorticoids are given [41].

Recently we reported that a 10-week period of 50% normal food intake followed by ad libitum feeding in female Sprague-Dawley rats initially 4 months or 15 to 16 months old extended the period of estrous cycles in the young rats and induced resumption of estrous cycles in the older rats [43]. After placement on ad libitum feeding, 100% of both age groups resumed cycling, the young rats for a much longer period than the older rats, and both groups continued to exhibit more cycles than their ad-libitum-fed controls. Apparently, this relatively brief period of underfeeding followed by refeeding increased the efficiency of the hypothalamic mechanisms regulating LH release. Thus, when rats were underfed for 10 weeks and then placed on ad libitum feeding and subsequently ovariectomized, the rise in LH secretion was greater in the old than in the young rats; also, when short-term underfed rats were fed ad libitum, subsequently ovariectomized, and given estradiol followed by progesterone to produce positive feedback, the old rats showed a greater rise in serum LH levels than the young rats [Quigley and Meites, unpubl. data]. These results provide evidence that even a relatively short period of underfeeding cannot only delay loss of estrous cycles in young rats approaching the end of their normal cycling period, but can also rejuvenate the neuroendocrine mechanisms regulating cycling in older rats and induce cycling. The temporary decrease in estrogen secretion during underfeeding, when the rats cease to cycle, may also reduce the damaging effects of estrogen on the neurons secreting GnRH and NE.

Conclusions

It is generally agreed that no current theory or hypothesis can explain all the possible causes for the decline in body functions with time. It is agreed that the major control of aging is exerted by the genome, but the question remains as to whether it operates at the level of individual cells or via the homeostatic and integrative systems of the body. Studies of isolated cells in vitro provide a method for assessing the role of intrinsic factors, including the molecular mechanisms involved in cellular function. However, under in vivo conditions, cells do not exist in isolation and are critically influenced by contiguous cells and by hormones, nutrients, waste products of metabolism, blood gases, acid-base balance, temperature ambience, hemodynamic changes, antibodies, etc. Furthermore, cells in vivo are subjected to environmental influences that operate via the neuroendocrine system. In rats, for example, stress stimulates the CNS to increase pituitary release of adrenocorticotropic hormone, PRL, and β-endorphin, and to decrease release of thyroid-stimulating hormone, GH, and gonadotropins. These alterations in hormone secretion, particularly when the stress is chronic, can alter cellular functions and aging processes. It is clear, therefore, that investigations of homeostatic and integrative mechanisms, particularly those of the neuroendocrine and immune systems, are essential for a full understanding of the causes of aging.

The most prominent theory of cellular aging was that advanced by Hayflick and Moorhead [44]. They noted that cultures of human fibroblasts in vitro had only a finite capacity to divide, and interpreted this as indicative of a basic change in genomic expression that occurs in all cells during aging. This can also be considered as an example of programed aging. Although this finding represents a landmark in gerontological research, and has been widely confirmed, it is difficult to apply it to aging of the neuroendocrine system, because (a) study of isolated neuroendocrine cells in vitro can provide only limited information on their homeostatic and integrative roles in vivo, (b) neurons of the brain do not divide since they are postmitotic cells, (c) damage and loss of neurons in the hypothalamus may be due to environmental agents as well as to a genomic program, and (d) despite damage or loss of neurons, there appear to be enough neurons remaining in the hypothalamus and enough cells in other neuroendocrine components of old rats to perform their functions when appropriately stimulated. The three aging decrements we have studied in the rat appear to be due mainly to lack of sufficient stimulation by CAs in the hypothalamus.

The various molecular theories of aging remain to be proven, and their possible relation to aging of the neuroendocrine system is unknown. The theory that there is an increase with age in DNA 'breaks' and a reduced ability to 'repair' these breaks has not been proven by experimental studies [45] and has not been investigated in neuroendocrine cells. Another theory states that errors develop in transfer of information from DNA via mRNA, resulting in errors in protein synthesis and cell death [46], but there is little evidence in support of this theory, and it does not appear to apply to neuroendocrine cells. There is no evidence that erroneous peptide hormones are produced by the hypothalamus of old rats, or that erroneous protein or peptide hormones are secreted by the pituitary or other endocrine tissues during aging. Although several hypothalamic and pituitary hormones have been shown to be present in different molecular weight forms, and the ratio of one form to another may change during aging, no new peptide or protein hormones have been found during aging.

We believe that the neuroendocrine approach can provide many answers to questions about the causes of aging in the rat, and perhaps in man. Many unsolved problems remain, particularly the role of the genome in the aging of the neuroendocrine system. To what extent is the genome responsible for the declines in hypothalamic, pituitary, and target gland functions? Are there limitations to the capacity of aging cells to respond to hormonal stimulation? How do the immune and neuroendocrine systems interact during aging? The demonstrations that correction of hypothalamic deficiencies can delay or reverse aging processes in rats point to the central role of the neuroendocrine system in the onset and progress of these processes. The importance of the neuroendocrine system in initiating aging changes is further emphasized when some of the same aging developments that normally occur in older rats can be experimentally reproduced in young rats by reducing hypothalamic CA activity. It can be concluded, therefore, that some of the declines in body functions in rats are not dependent on *age* per se, but on specific changes in hypothalamic function. We believe that it may even be possible, by neuroendocrine intervention, to maintain estrous cycles, inhibit development of mammary and pituitary tumors, and elevate GH secretion and protein synthesis practically to the end of life in rats. Whether this would alter the length of their life is unknown, but chronic administration of *L*-dopa was reported to lengthen the life span of mice [47]. It is clear that the neuroendocrine system is critically involved in initiating and advancing the decline in body functions during life.

References

1 Meites, J.; Goya, R.; Takahashi, S.: Why the neuroendocrine system is important in aging processes. Exp. Gerontol. *22:* 1–15 (1987).

2 Aschheim, P.: Aging in the hypothalamic-hypophyseal ovarian axis in the rat; in Everitt, Burgess, Hypothalamus, pituitary and aging, pp. 376–418 (Thomas, Springfield 1976).

3 Peng, M.: Changes in hormone uptake and receptors in the hypothalamus during aging; in Meites, Neuroendocrinology of aging, pp. 61–72 (Plenum Press, New York 1983).

4 Peng, M.: Aging of hypothalamic-pituitary ovarian function. Fert. Steril. *23:* 535–542 (1972).

5 Shaar, C.; Euker, J.; Riegle, G.; Meites, J.: Effects of castration and gonadal steroids on serum luteinizing hormone and prolactin in old and young rats. J. Endocr. *66:* 45–51 (1975).

6 Wise, P.; Ratner, A.: Effects of ovariectomy on plasma LH, FSH, estradiol, and progesterone and medial basal hypothalamic LHRH concentrations in old and young rats. Neuroendocrinology *30:* 15–19 (1980).
7 Steger, R.; Huang, H.; Meites, J.: Relation of aging to hypothalamic LHRH content and serum gonadal steroids in female rats. Proc. Soc. exp. Biol. Med. *161:* 251–254 (1979).
8 Pekary, A.; Carlson, H.; Yamada, B.; Sharp, P.; Walfish, P.; Hershman, J.: Thyrotropin-releasing hormone levels decrease in hypothalamus of aging rats. Neurobiol. Aging *5:* 221–226 (1984).
9 Pekary, A.; Mirell, C.; Turner, L.; Walfish, P.; Hershman, J.: Hypothalamic secretion of thyrotropin releasing hormone declines in aging rats. J. Geront. *42:* 447–450 (1987).
10 Sonntag, W.; Gottschall, P.; Meites, J.: Increased secretion of somatostatin-28 from hypothalamic neurons of aged rats in vitro. Brain Res. *380:* 229–234 (1986).
11 Simpkins, J.; Mueller, G.; Huang, H.; Meites, J.: Evidence for depressed catecholamine and enhanced serotonin metabolism in aging male rats: possible relation to gonadotropin secretion. Endocrinology *100:* 1672–1678 (1977).
12 Wise, P.: Aging of the female reproductive system. Rev. Bio. Res. Aging *1:* 195–222 (1983).
13 Martin, J.: Brain regulation of growth hormone secretion, in Martini, Ganong, Frontiers in neuroendocrinology, vol. 4, pp. 129–168 (Raven Press, New York 1976).
14 Gudelsky, A.; Nansel, D.; Porter, J.: Dopaminergic control of prolactin secretion in the aging male rat. Brain Res. *204:* 446–450 (1981).
15 Simpkins, J.: Regional changes in monoamine metabolism in the aging constant estrous rat. Neurobiol. Aging *4:* 3309–3314 (1984).
16 Watkins, B.; Meites, J.; Riegle, G.: Age-related changes in pituitary responsiveness to LHRH in female rats. Endocrinology *97:* 543–548 (1975).
17 Sonntag, W.; Forman, L.; Fiori, J.; Hylka, V.; Meites, J.: Decreased ability of old male rats to secrete luteinizing hormone (LH) is not due to alterations in pituitary LH-releasing hormone receptors. Endocrinology *114:* 1657–1664 (1984).
18 Harman, S.; Talbert, G.: Reproductive aging; in Finch, Schneider, Handbook of the biology of aging; 2nd ed., pp. 457–510 (Van Nostrand & Reinhold, New York 1985).
19 Roth, G.: Altered hormone/neurotransmitter action during aging: receptor and post-receptor changes; in Roy, Chatterjee, Molecular basis of aging, pp. 167–186 (Academic Press, New York 1984).
20 Hylka, V.; Sonntag, W.; Meites, J.: Reduced ability of old male rats to release ACTH and corticosterone in response to CRF administration. Proc. Soc. exp. Biol. Med. *175:* 1–4 (1984).
21 Takahashi, S.; Meites, J.: GH binding to liver in young and old female rats: relation to somatomedin-C secretion. Proc. Soc. exp. Biol. Med. *186:* 229–233 (1987).
22 Takahashi, S.; Gottschall, P.; Quigley, K.; Goya, R.; Meites, J.: Growth hormone secretory patterns in young, middle-aged and old female rats. Neuroendocrinology *46:* 137–142 (1987).
23 Greenspan, F.; Li, C.; Simpson, M.; Evans, H.: Growth hormone; in Emmens, Hormone assay, pp. 273–290 (Academic Press, New York 1950).

24 Florini, J.; Roberts, S.: Effects of rat age on blood levels of somatomedin-like growth factors. J. Geront. *35:* 23–30 (1980).

25 Shock, N.: Systemic integration; in Finch, Hayflick, Handbook of the biology of aging, pp. 639–665 (Van Nostrand & Reinhold, New York 1977).

26 Clemens, J.; Amenomori, Y.; Jenkins, T.; Meites, J.: Effects of hypothalamic stimulation, hormones and drugs on ovarian function in old female rats. Proc. Soc. exp. Biol. Med. *132:* 561–563 (1969).

27 Welsch, C.; Ayslworth, C.: Relation of the neuroendocrine system to the development of mammary tumors in rats during aging; in Meites, Neuroendocrinology of aging, pp. 333–352 (Plenum, New York 1983).

28 Furth, J.: Hormones as etiological agents in neoplasia; in Becker, Cancer, pp. 75–120 (Plenum, New York 1975).

29 Brawer, J.; Naftolin, F.; Martin, J.; Sonnenschein, C.: Effects of a single injection of estradiol valerate on the hypothalamic arcuate nucleus and on reproductive function in the female rat. Endocrinology *103:* 501–512 (1978).

30 Sarkar, D.; Gottschall, P.; Meites, J.: Damage to hypothalamic dopaminergic neurons is associated with development of prolactin-secreting pituitary tumors. Science *218:* 684–686 (1982).

31 Finch, C.; Felicio, L.; Mobbs, C.; Nelson, J.: Ovarian and steroidal influences on neuroendocrine aging processes in female rodents. Endocr. Rev. *5:* 467–497 (1984).

32 Sarkar, D.; Gottschall, P.; Meites, J.: Decline of tuberoinfundibular dopaminergic function resulting from chronic hyperprolactinemia in rats. Endocrinology *115:* 1269–1274 (1984).

33 Landfield, P.; Waymire, J.; Lynch, G.: Hippocampal aging and adrenocorticoids: quantitative correlations. Science *202:* 1098–1102 (1978).

34 Kurz, E.; Sengelaub, D.; Arnold, A.: Androgens regulate the dendritic length of mammalian motoneurons in adulthood. Science *232:* 395–398 (1986).

35 Sar, M.: Estradiol is concentrated in tyrosine hydroxylase-containing neurons of the hypothalamus. Science *223:* 938–940 (1984).

36 Benedetti, M.; Dank, H.; Dostert, P.: Age-related changes in brain MAO and in enzymes involved in detoxication process of MAO-generated compounds; in Biaggio, Spano, Toffano, Gessa, Modulation of central and peripheral transmitter function, pp. 255–267 (Liviana, Padova 1986).

37 Strehler, B.: Time, cells, and aging, pp. 5–30 (Academic Press, New York 1985).

38 Masoro, E.: Nutrition as a modulator of the aging process. Physiologist *27:* 98–101 (1984).

39 Wurtman, R.; Wurtman, J.: Nutrition and the brain, vol. 2 (Raven Press, New York 1983).

40 Campbell, G.; Kurcz, M.; Marshall, S.; Meites, J.: Effects of starvation in rats on serum levels of follicle stimulating hormone, luteinizing hormone, thyrotropin, growth hormone and prolactin: response to LH-releasing hormone and thyrotropin-releasing hormone. Endocrinology *100:* 580–587 (1977).

41 Everitt, A.: Hypophysectomy and aging in the rat; in Everitt, Burgess, Hypothalamus, pituitary and aging, pp. 68–85 (Thomas, Springfield 1976).

42 Everitt, A.: The neuroendocrine system and aging. Gerontology *26:* 108–119 (1980).

43 Quigley, K.; Goya, R.; Meites, J.: Rejuvenating effects of 10-week underfeeding period on estrous cycles in young and old rats. Neurobiol. Aging *8:* 225–232 (1987).
44 Hayflick, L.; Moorhead, P.: The serial cultivation of human diploid cell strains. Expl Cell Res. *25:* 585–621 (1961).
45 Williams, J.; Dearfield, K.: DNA damage and repair; in Florini, Handbook of biochemistry in aging, pp. 25–48 (CRC Press, Boca Raton 1981).
46 Orgel, L.: The maintenance of the accuracy of protein synthesis and its relevance to aging. Proc. natn. Acad. Sci *49:* 517–521 (1963).
47 Cotzias, G.; Miller, S.; Nicholson, A., Jr.; Matson, W.; Tang, L.: Levodopa, fertility, and longevity. Proc. natn. Acad. Sci *71:* 2466–2469 (1974).

Dr. Joseph Meites, Department of Physiology, Michigan State University,
East Lansing, MI 48824-1101 (USA)

Interdiscipl. Topics Geront., vol. 24, pp. 51–60 (Karger, Basel 1988)

Hormonal Basis of Aging: Antiaging Action of Hypophysectomy

Arthur V. Everitt

Department of Geriatric Medicine, University of Sydney, Repatriation General Hospital, Concord, Australia

The concept of aging as a hormone deficiency condition had its beginnings with the spectacular announcement by Brown-Sequard [1] in Paris in 1889 that he at age 72 was rejuvenated by an animal testicular extract. In later studies during the early years of the 20th century aging was attributed to a deficiency of hormones from the thyroid and anterior pituitary and in the 1960s age-associated bone loss in women was related to estrogen deficiency [2].

The idea that pituitary and adrenocortical hormones have aging actions arose in the 1930s from clinical studies [3] showing premature aging in patients with Cushing's syndrome. In the 1950s and 1960s many workers demonstrated aging actions of hormones in a variety of rodent tissues [4–11], and thereby established hormones as causal factors in aging. Since the 1960s researchers have been investigating central mechanisms of aging [7, 12–16], and have demonstrated damaging actions of steroid hormones on the hypothalamus [15] and hippocampus [16].

Hormonal-Nutritional Interaction

Many studies of hormone action on aging phenomena are complicated by changes in food intake and metabolism. In the rat, food intake is increased by thyroid hormone, growth hormone, corticosteroids and insulin [11, 17, 18] and decreased by thyroidectomy [11] and hypophysectomy [8]. Conversely long term undernutrition in man and rodents is accompanied by low circulating levels of hormones secreted by the anterior pituitary, thyroid, testis and ovary [18]. Consequently many hormonal studies of aging need to consider this hormonal-nutritional interaction. For example, thyroxine increases the aging rate in tail tendon collagen in proportion to the rise in food intake, but if food intake is restricted thyroxine does not increase the aging rate [11]. Many of the aging effects attributed to hormones may be due to actions of dietary factors or products of food metabolism, e.g. glucose has an aging action on tissue proteins [19].

Hypophysectomy in the Rat

Hypophysectomy has an anti-aging action in many tissues, including reduced morphological aging of the target glands, thyroid (tumors), adrenal cortex (age pigment), ovary (oocyte loss) and testis (tumors). Early workers had shown that the normal rate of oocyte loss with age from mouse ovary is halved by hypophysectomy at age 40–50 days [6]. Ovaries from these middle-aged hypophysectomized mice when grafted into young ovariectomized mice are able to release ova which after fertilization give rise to normal litters, at an age when ovaries from intact controls are sterile.

Most hypophysectomy studies have been concerned with aging in non-endocrine organs. In studies on male Wistar rats where food intake is controlled hypophysectomy at age 50–70 days with little or no cortisone therapy has been found to have a greater antiaging action than food restriction begun at the same age [20]. The tensile strength of rat tail tendon collagen fibers increases markedly with age; this increase is halved by hypophysectomy and reduced by 30% in food-restricted rats where both groups have the same food intake [20]. Using the same experimental design hypophysectomy had a greater inhibitory action on thickening of the glomerular basement membrane [21] and the thoracic aorta [22]. Hypophysectomy also had a greater inhibitory action on the development of age-associated diseases, including the incidence of glomerular disease and proteinaceous casts in kidney [20], incidence of hind leg paralysis in very old rats [23] and the incidence of tumors in old rats [22]. Tumors of the thyroid, adrenal and testis were found in 48% of old controls but only in 3% of hypophysectomized rats older than 800 days [22]. Gross pathology was seen at autopsy in 100% of male controls aged 800 days or more but in only 74% of food-restricted and 48% of hypophysectomized rats [24]. The lower incidence of pathology in old age may be related to the retarded aging of the immune system in long-term hypophysectomy in rodents. Compared with controls hypophysectomy in the rat improves the rejection of xenografts [25] and enhances the response to immunization with sheep erythrocytes [26] and in the mouse delays thymic involution [27]. The immune and neuroendocrine systems appear to interact [28].

When housed under good conditions in a warm room at 27 °C the male hypophysectomized rat is healthier in old age and lives longer than intact controls, even when receiving no replacement therapy. Using the transauricular technique and weekly subcutaneous injection of 1 mg cortisone acetate hypophysectomy at 60 days prolonged the mean life duration to 925 days compared with 858 days in food-restricted rats on the same food intake and 785 days for ad-libitum-fed controls. The maximum life durations recorded from studies over a period of 25 years are 1,201 days for ad-libitum-fed controls, 1,525 days for food-restricted rats and 1,335 days for hypophysectomized rats [29]. Thus food restriction is better than hypophysectomy in prolonging life, probably because the optimal hormone replacement therapy for survival of hypophysectomized rats is not yet known.

Aging Action of Hormones

It was postulated by Everitt [13] in 1973 that 'most hormones accelerate aging processes in their target organs'. There is now a large literature showing that hormones have aging effects in many different tissues. For example, in the hypothalamic-pituitary-ovarian axis there is evidence that the normal regulatory hormones (estrogens and gonadotropins) have aging effects in their target cells (fig. 1). Chronic estrogen therapy has been shown to damage the arcuate nucleus in the hypothalamus [15], while hypophysectomy by eliminating gonadotropin secretion, slows the loss of oocytes from the ovary of the mouse [6].

Age-related changes affected by hormones range through loss of receptors [16], cytological damage [14, 16, 21], cell loss [21], enzyme changes [30], cross-linking of collagen [9, 11], arteriosclerosis [10], glomerulosclerosis in kidney [20, 21], tumorigenesis and tumor growth [22, 31].

Since the aging actions of hormones have been reviewed previously [32, 33] only a summary is given here with reference to recent studies. The effects of pituitary hormones on aging of their targets in the thyroid, adrenal cortex, ovary and testis have received little attention in recent years. There is no doubt that at puberty in both sexes the large rise in gonadotro-

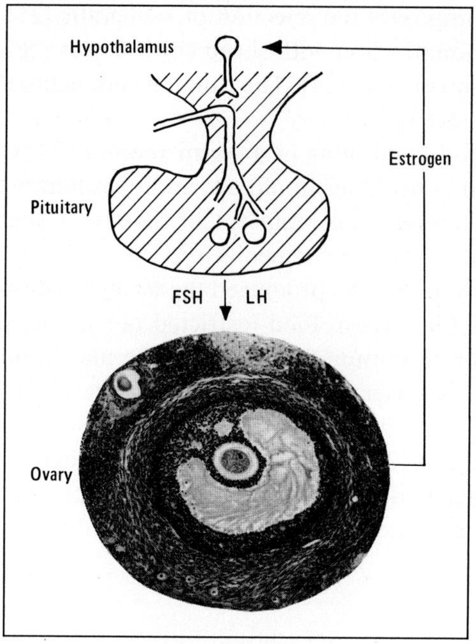

Fig. 1. The hormonal basis of aging in the hypothalamic-pituitary-ovarian axis. Hypophysectomy, which removes the source of gonadotropins (follicle-stimulating hormone, FSH, and luteinizing hormone, LH), halves the life-long rate of oocyte loss from the ovary of three different strains of mice [6]. Long-term estrogen therapy accelerates, while chronic ovariectomy delays age-related degenerative changes in the hypothalamic arcuate nucleus of rats and mice [15]. The arcuate nucleus is involved in the secretion of gonadotropin-releasing hormone. In this way pituitary gonadotropins appear to accelerate ovarian aging, while estrogens increase aging in the receptor cells of the arcuate nucleus of the hypothalamus. Thus the hormones which control the normal operation of this axis also appear to modulate its aging.

pin secretion activates the gonads, but the specific timing mechanism is poorly understood and probably involves central inhibition [34]. Early studies found that unilateral ovariectomy in the mouse, which increases gonadotropin secretion, shortened the reproductive life of the remaining ovary [35]. Similarly partial thyroidectomy, which increases thyrotropin secretion, causes a premature development of tumors in the remaining thyroid tissue [36].

Adrenocortical hormones and stress have been associated with accelerated aging in a number of studies [10, 16, 37]. The hyperadrenocorticoid state of Cushing's disease is characterized by a number of metabolic and pathophysiological changes (diabetes mellitus, hyperlipidemia, hypertension, osteoporosis, immunosuppression, arteriosclerosis and muscle wasting) which are commonly seen in older patients. In the rat glucocorticoids and stress have been shown to increase the aging of tail tendon collagen, produce an early onset of arteriosclerosis [10], lead to senescent changes in the hippocampus such as loss of receptors, neuronal degeneration and death [16, 37].

Estrogen in the rat and mouse has a long-term effect on the brain causing a neuroendocrine syndrome of reproductive aging characterized by changes in the hypothalamus (glial hypertrophy in the arcuate nucleus, decrease in catecholamine content), pituitary (increased dopamine, impaired luteinizing hormone surge) and ovary (loss of cycling) [15]. These changes are attenuated by ovariectomy in the young rodent [15]. Estrogens have been implicated in the growth of pituitary tumors [15] and, via increased prolactin secretion, the production of mammary tumors [38].

Androgens, when administered to rats neonatally, masculinize the hypothalamus with regard to the secretory pattern of gonadotropins at puberty [39]. Benign prostatic hypertrophy does not develop in men castrated prepubertally [40], thus implicating androgens in this age-related disease. Interestingly the adrenal androgen, dehydroepiandrostenedione, has an antiaging action in rodents because it diminishes tumor incidence, diabetes, obesity and proteinuria development [41].

Thyroxine administered neonatally to rats damages the hypothalamic thyroid-stimulating-hormone controlling mechanism [42]. Such rats become hypothyroid and like hypophysectomized rats have increased life duration whereas chronic hyperthyroidism in adult rats shortens life [42]. Thyroid hormones are known to have maturation effects on the brain [43] and skeleton [4]. Thyroxine accelerates the aging of tail tendon collagen [11] and increases the incidence of age-related kidney lesions. Thyroidectomy retards collagen aging [11] and renal age pathology.

Growth hormone is reported to promote skeletal aging [32], increase the incidence of age-related renal pathology and tumors in many tissues and to thicken capillary basement membranes [44], an age-related change. Hypophysectomy greatly reduces the incidence of renal disease [20–22] and tumors [22, 24] and slows age-related thickening of the glomerular basement membrane [21].

High circulating prolactin levels in old rats [45] may be associated with some age-related changes such as mammary tumor development [31,

38] as already mentioned. Prolactin is reported to damage the retina and dopaminergic neurons [45]. Old hypophysectomized male Wistar rats in our University of Sydney colony do not develop mammary tumors, whereas 8% of controls older than 800 days carry these tumors [unpubl. data].

Hormonal Molecular Mechanisms of Aging

Hormonal effects on aging at the molecular level are poorly understood. Since genetic factors play a major role in aging, studies of the effect of hormones on gene expression are essential to understanding the nature of aging.

At the target cell the hormone must first combine with a receptor before interacting with the genome, enzymes, etc. In many tissues there is a loss of hormone receptors with increasing age [46], which in the case of glucocorticoid receptors may be due to the cumulative effects of repeated stress and hypersecretion of glucocorticoids [16, 37].

According to Kanungo [47] the main phases in life (differentiation, growth, reproduction and senescence) may be due to the sequential activation and repression of genes by gene products, including hormones. Gene expression is the basis of differentiation and development in early life, and there is no doubt that hormones affect gene expression. Are the age changes in gene expression in later life due to the long-term effects of hormones?

Aging produces a decline in gene expression, both in transcription (nuclear RNA synthesis) and translation (protein synthesis) in a wide variety of tissues and organs [48]. The expression of genes for specific enzymes can be stimulated acutely by hormones [49]. Liver nuclear RNA synthesis is inhibited by acute hypophysectomy, thyroidectomy or castration and restored by growth hormone, thyroxine and testosterone [49]. As with a number of other functions [20–27] long-term hypophysectomy is able to minimize the age-associated decline in liver nuclear RNA synthesis [50]. Thus long-term hypophysectomy is able to retard this age-associated decline in gene expression. Factors contributing to the loss of gene expression [51] may be (a) change in genetic program, (b) coding error or point mutation in DNA, (c) impaired control of transcription and posttranscription, (d) reduced transport of RNA and (e) protein missynthesis. The effect of hormones on these factors is largely unknown.

Hypothalamic-Pituitary Regulation of Aging

It has been shown that long-term hypophysectomy like food restriction slows the rate of physiological aging in collagen, decreases the decline in protein synthesis, preserves immunocompetence in old age, reduces the incidence of age pathology and prolongs life.

Pituitary hormones and food factors are clearly involved in promoting the rate of aging in many tissues. A third factor in aging is tissue temperature, a well-known determinant of aging in insects [52]; the aging of tail-tendon collagen is slower when tail temperature is low [53]. These three functions, pituitary hormone secretion, feeding behavior and body temperature, are regulated by specific areas in the hypothalamus, which in turn receive inputs from higher centers such as the hippocampus, amygdala, pineal, etc. Several studies have implicated the hippocampus [16, 37] and pineal [54] as playing a role in aging. It is possible for environmental factors, such as stress, diet, temperature, microorganisms, hormones, metabolites and drugs, by acting on the hypothalamus and higher centers to modulate this central regulation of aging through the hypothalamic-pituitary-endocrine axis.

References

1 Brown-Sequard, C.E.: Seconde note sur les effets produits chez l'homme par des injections sous-cutanées d'un liquide retiré des testicules frais de cobaye et de chien, C.r. Séanc. Soc. Biol. 9e sér. *1:* 420 (1889).

2 Davis, M.E.; Strandfjord, J.M.; Langl, L.H.: Estrogens and the aging process. The detection, prevention and retardation of osteoporosis. J. Am. med. Ass. *196:* 219–224 (1966).

3 Raab, W.: Analogien zwischen gewissen Alterserscheinungen und der Cushingschen Krankheit. Wien. klin. Wschr. *49:* 112–113 (1936).

4 Asling, C.W.; Simpson, M.E.; Li, C.H.; Evans, H.M.: The effects of chronic administration of thyroxine to hypophysectomized rats on their skeletal growth, maturation and response to growth hormone. Anat. Rec. *119:* 101–117 (1954).

5 Everitt, A.V.: The effect of prolonged thyroxine treatment on the aging male rat. Gerontologia *3:* 37–54 (1959).

6 Jones, E.C.; Krohn, P.L.: The effect of hypophysectomy on age changes in the ovaries of mice. J. Endocr. *21:* 497–509 (1961).

7 Aschheim, P.: Résultats fournis par le greffe hétérochrone des ovaires dans l'étude de la régulation hypothalamo-hypophyso-ovarienne de la rate sénile. Gerontologia *10:* 65–75 (1964/1965).

8 Everitt, A.V.; Cavanagh, L.M.: The ageing process in the hypophysectomized rat. Gerontologia *11:* 198–207 (1965).

9 Verzár, F.; Spichtin, H.: The role of the pituitary in the aging of collagen. Gerontologia *12:* 48–56 (1965).

10 Wexler, B.C.; Kittinger, G.W.: Adrenocortical function in arteriosclerotic female breeder rats. J. Atheroscler. Res. *5:* 317–329 (1965).

11 Giles, J.S.; Everitt, A.V.: The role of thyroid and food intake in the ageing of collagen fibres I. In the young rat. Gerontologia *13:* 65–69 (1967).

12 Dilman, V.M.: Age-associated elevation of hypothalamic threshold to feedbank control and its role in development, ageing and disease. Lancet *i:* 1211–1219 (1971).

13 Everitt, A.V.: The hypothalamic-pituitary control of aging and age related pathology. Exp. Gerontol. *8:* 265–277 (1973).

14 Timiras, P.S.; Choy, V.J.; Hudson, D.B.: Neuroendocrine pacemaker for growth, development and ageing. Age Ageing *11:* 73–88 (1982).

15 Finch, C.E.; Felicio, L.S.; Mobbs, C.V.; Nelson, J.F.: Ovarian and steroidal influences on neuroendocrine aging processes in female rodents. Endocr. Rev. *5:* 467–497 (1984).

16 Sapolsky, R.M; Krey, L.C.; McEwen, B.S.: The neuroendocrinology of stress and aging: the glucocorticoid cascade hypothesis. Endocr. Rev. *7:* 284–301 (1986).

17 York, D.A.; Bray, G.A.: Dependence of hypothalamic obesity on insulin, the pituitary and adrenal gland. Endocrinology *90:* 885–894 (1972).

18 Everitt, A.V.; Porter, B.: Nutrition and aging; in Everitt, Burgess, Hypothalamus, pituitary and aging, pp. 570–613 (Thomas, Springfield 1976).

19 Cerami, A.H.; Brownlee, M.: Glucose and aging. Scient. Am. *256:* 82–88 (1987).

20 Everitt, A.V.; Wyndham, J.R.; Barnard, D.L.: The anti-aging action of hypophysectomy in hypothalamic obese rats: effects on collagen aging, age-associated proteinuria development and renal histopathology. Mech. Age. Dev. *22:* 233–251 (1983).

21 Wyndham, J.R.; Everitt, A.V.; Major, J.: Inhibitory effect of hypophysectomy and food restriction on glomerular basement membrane thickening, proteinuria and renal enlargement in aging male Wistar rats. Archs Geront. Geriatr. *6:* 323–337 (1987).

22 Everitt, A.V.; Seedsman, N.J.; Jones, F.: The effects of hypophysectomy and continuous food restriction begun at ages 70 and 400 days, on collagen aging, proteinuria, incidence of pathology and longevity in the male rat. Mech. Age. Dev. *12:* 161–172 (1980).

23 Everitt, A.V.; Shorey, C.D.; Ficarra, M.A.: Skeletal muscle aging in the hind limb of the old male Wistar rat: inhibitory effect of hypophysectomy and food restriction. Archs Geront. Geriatr. *4:* 101–115 (1985).

24 Everitt, A.V.: Nutrition, hormones and aging. Chulalongkorn Med. J. *29:* 863–872 (1985).

25 Bilder, G.E.; Denckla, W.D.: Restoration of ability to reject xenografts and clear carbon after hypophysectomy of adult rats. Mech. Age. Dev. *8:* 152–163 (1977).

26 Scott, M.; Bolla, R.; Denckla, W.D.: Age-related changes in immune function of rats and the effect of long-term hypophysectomy. Mech. Age. Dev. *11:* 127–136 (1979).

27 Harrison, D.E.; Archer, J.R.; Astle, C.M.: The effect of hypophysectomy on thymic aging in mice. J. Immun. *129:* 2673–2677 (1982).

28 Blalock, J.E.; Smith, E.M.: A complete regulatory loop between the immune and neuroendocrine systems. Fed. Proc. *44:* 108–111 (1985).

29 Everitt, A.V.; Wyndham, J.R.: Hypothalamic-pituitary regulation and aging; in Adelman, Roth, Endocrine and neuroendocrine mechanisms of aging, pp. 123–165 (CRC Press, Boca Raton 1982).
30 Kanungo, M.S.: Biochemistry of aging, pp. 79–128 (Academic Press, London 1980).
31 Blask, D.E.; Leadem, C.A.: Neuroendocrine aspects of neoplastic growth – a review. Neuroendocr. Lett. *9:* 1–11 (1987).
32 Everitt, A.V.: Pituitary function and aging; in Danon, Shock, Aging – a challenge to science and policy, pp. 249–266 (Oxford University Press, Oxford 1981).
33 Everitt, A.V.: The genetic clock-hormone theory of aging; in Preston, Biological and social aspects of mortality and length of life, pp. 279–301 (Ordina, Liège 1982).
34 Reiter, E.O.; Grumbach, M.M.: Neuroendocrine control mechanisms and the onset of puberty. A. Rev. Physiol. *44:* 595–613 (1982).
35 Jones, E.C.; Krohn, P.L.: The effect of unilateral ovariectomy on the reproductive life span of mice. J. Endocr. *20:* 129–134 (1960).
36 Doniach, I.; Williams, E.D.: The development of thyroid and pituitary tumours in the rat two years after partial thyroidectomy. Br. J. Cancer *16:* 222–231 (1962).
37 Landfield, P.; Waymire, J.; Lynch, G.: Hippocampal aging and adrenocorticoids: a quantitative correlation. Science *202:* 1098–1102 (1978).
38 Ito, A.; Naito, M.; Watanabe, H.; Yokoro, K.: Prolactin and aging: X-irradiated and estrogen-induced rat mammary carcinogenesis. J. natn. Cancer Inst. *73:* 123–126 (1984).
39 Dormer, G.: Sexual differentiation of the brain. Vitams. Horm. *38:* 325–381 (1980).
40 Moore, R.A.: An endocrinology of neoplastic disease, p. 194 (Oxford University Press, New York 1947).
41 Pashko, L.L.; Fairman, D.K.; Schwartz, A.G.: Inhibition of proteinuria development in aging Sprague-Dawley rats and C57BL/6 mice by long-term treatment with dehydroepiandrosterone. J. Geront. *41:* 433–438 (1986).
42 Ooka, H.; Shinkai, T.: Effects of chronic hyperthyroidism on the lifespan of the rat. Mech. Age. Dev. *33:* 275–282 (1986).
43 Dussault, J.H.; Ruel, J.: Thyroid hormones and brain development. A. Rev. Physiol. *49:* 321–334 (1987).
44 Oikawa, S.; Maruhama, Y.; Goto, Y.: Evidence for direct effect of growth hormone on capillary basement membrane thickness. Tohoku J. exp. Med. *46:* 167–174 (1985).
45 Sarkar, D.K.; Gottschall, P.E.; Meites, J.: Decline of tuberoinfundibular dopaminergic function resulting from chronic hyperprolactinemia in rats. Endocrinology *115:* 1269–1274 (1984).
46 Roth, G.S.: Hormone receptor changes during adulthood and senescence: significance for aging research. Fed. Proc. *38:* 1910–1914 (1979).
47 Kanungo, M.S.: A model for ageing. J. theor. Biol. *53:* 253–1961 (1975).
48 Richardson, A.; Cheung, H.T.: Current concepts. I. The relationship between age-related changes in gene expression, protein turnover and the responsiveness of an organism to stimuli. Life. Sci. *31:* 605–613 (1982).
49 Windnell, C.C.; Tata, J.R.: Additive effects of thyroid hormone, growth hormone and testosterone on deoxyribonucleic acid-dependent ribonucleic acid polymerase in rat liver nuclei. Biochem. J. *98:* 621–629 (1966).

50 Bolla, R.; Denckla, W.D.: Effect of hypophysectomy on liver nuclear ribonucleic acid synthesis in aging rats. Biochem. J. *184:* 669–674 (1979).
51 Muller, W.; Agutter, P.S.; Bernd, A.; Bachmann, M.; Schroder, H.C.: Role of post-transcriptional events in aging: consequences for gene expression in eukaryotic cells; in Bergener, Ermini, Stahelin, Thresholds in aging, pp. 21–57 (Academic Press, London 1985).
52 Hollingsworth, M.J.: Temperature and length of life in Drosophila. Exp. Gerontol. *4:* 49–55 (1969).
53 Everitt, A.V.; Porter, B.D.; Steele, M.: Dietary, caging and temperature factors in the ageing of collagen fibres in rat tail tendon. Gerontology *27:* 37–41 (1981).
54 Dilman, V.M.; Anisimov, V.N.; Ostroumova, M.N.; Khavinson, V.K.; Morozov, V.G.: Increase in lifespan of rats following polypeptide pineal extract treatment. Exp. Pathol. *17:* 539–545 (1979).

Dr. A.V. Everitt, Department of Geriatric Medicine, Ward 29, Concord Hospital, Concord, NSW 2139 (Australia)

Interdiscipl. Topics Geront., vol. 24, pp. 61–73 (Karger, Basel 1988)

Dietary Restriction and the Neuroendocrinology of Aging

B.J. Merry, Anne M. Holehan
Wolfson Institute, University of Hull, UK

It has been clearly established in a number of different experimental designs that the rate of aging, at least in rodent species, is amenable to manipulation by dietary means [1]. A 36–42% extension of maximum life span can be achieved in rats and mice by limiting access to their normal diet from weaning so as to maintain their growth rate at approximately 50% that of fully fed age-matched controls. This simple approach to restricted feeding is but one of many experimental strategies which has been employed to induce caloric restriction and enhanced longevity in rodents. Alternate day feeding and fasting regimes and ad libitum feeding of diets reduced either in protein or carbohydrate content have also been shown to extend longevity in rodent species. The molecular mechanism whereby calorie or dietary restriction can modify physiological aging and extend life span has not been determined. The suggestion has been made, however, that the process of aging may be under neural and endocrine control in a manner similar to development, growth and maturation [2].

Neuroendocrine Response to Dietary Restriction

The neuroendocrine system is known to regulate, to a greater or lesser degree, cellular metabolism in all tissues of the body, providing a critical link between the expression of the genetic program and its modification by environmental influences. Many attempts to explain the action of diet on longevity have invoked a role for the neuroendocrine system, beginning with the simple ideas derived from the work of McCay et al. [3] through to the complex hypotheses of Segall [2] and Meites et al. [4]. Further support for this idea is drawn from the extensive studies of Everitt et al. [5], in which they developed the use of early surgical hypophysectomy coupled to hormone replacement therapy in rats to retard aging and extend life span. Everitt and Porter [6] have further shown that food restriction, under certain conditions, will reduce the secretion of many anterior pituitary hormones, while Campbell et al. [7] have demonstrated that very severe underfeeding will decrease the production of hypothalamic releasing hormones.

The relationship between the antiaging actions of hypophysectomy and food restriction is unclear. Shortened survival times have been reported for hypophysectomized mice despite an apparent increase in motor activity and a more youthful appearance, these being designated as biomarkers of aging [8]. Less severe regimes of underfeeding than utilized by McCay et al. [3] have produced greater survival in terms of both mean and maximum life span for rats than achieved by surgical hypophysectomy. It is feasible, therefore, that surgical hypophysectomy is an alternative means of inducing chronic underfeeding in the rat.

A third approach to enhancing survival in rats has been developed by Segall et al. [9]. Rats were maintained on a diet which was fed ad libitum but was deficient in the amino acid, tryptophan. In general terms the effects induced by such a dietary regime are similar to those produced by severe food restriction, in that both growth and development are severely retarded and there is a delayed onset of reproductive senescence and tumor appearance when animals are returned to a balanced diet. Dietary tryptophan is the sole source of serotonin in the rat and in rats maintained on a tryptophan-deficient diet decreased brain serotonin levels are recorded [10]. Thus it can be argued that a pathway exists whereby dietary levels of essential amino acids can directly modify the activity of the monoaminergic neural pathways in the hypothalamus, leading to changes in the neuroendocrine system. Similarly the synthesis of acetylcholine can be enhanced by increasing the level in the brain of its precursor, choline, and the synthesis and release of dopamine and norepinephrine are modified by the dietary levels of their precursor, the amino acid tyrosine.

Segall [2] has argued that the neuroendocrine axis provides an intricate control of gene expression which is central to the ontogenetic processes and that senescence may be under similar neural and endocrine controls. Thus dietary restriction can be envisaged to operate through a complex neuroendocrine response mediated by monoamine transmitters in the hypothalamus, the synthesis and turnover of which are responding directly to serum concentrations of essential amino acids. It should be noted, however, that tryptophan is often the amino acid of lowest concentration in rodent diets and has been demonstrated to play a key role in protein synthesis by regulating the polysome profile [11]. In the tryptophan-restricted model the possibility exists that it is the direct effect on protein synthesis which is of prime importance rather than a shift in the neuroendocrine balance. In the following sections we will discuss the data which supports or contradicts a neuroendocrine basis for the action of dietary restriction.

Neurology

Anatomical evidence for a delayed rate of aging in neural tissue of dietary-restricted rodents has been published. Underfeeding Charles River CD rats reduced the age-related loss of pineal cells and resulted in the retention of a more juvenile-type pineal gland. The functional consequences of these observations in relation to the neuroendocrine system are unknown [12, 13].

The imposition of restricted feeding by alternate day fasting and feeding has been shown to substantially retard the loss of striatal dopamine receptors which are known to be responsible for altered dopaminergic control of specific physiological and behavioral functions in senescent rats [14]. There is strong evidence to link dopamine receptor loss, motor behavioral performance and stereotypic behavior in aged animals [15]. It has been demonstrated that reduced striatal receptor loss which appears to be a chronic effect of underfeeding rather than an acute response, can be translated into a selective reduction of some of the motor behavioral deficits associated with senescence. Following unilateral lesioning in the left substantia nigra with 6-OH dopamine, old (24–26 month) dietary-restricted animals responded as well as 6-month ad-libitum-fed rats, and significantly better than 24-month-old ad-libitum-fed rats to combinations of amphetamine, or the cholinergic inhibitor, atropine, when injected directly into the right caudate nucleus [15].

This finding has been replicated and extended in a study using ^3H spiperone as the ligand in the analysis of striatal dopamine receptors [16]. Further observations of the neurochemistry of the alternate day feeding model of retarded aging in rats have demonstrated a markedly higher density of striatal muscarinic binding sites and higher activities of cerebellar, hippocampal and striatal choline acetyltransferase in old restricted rats when compared with their ad-libitum fed counterparts. Conversely, *L*-glutamic acid decarboxylase and tyrosine hydroxylase levels in the corpus striatum, cerebral cortex, hippocampus and cerebellum were relatively unaffected by the restricted feeding regime.

The changes in brain neurochemistry in the dietary-restricted rat appear to be a chronic rather than an acute response resulting in a selective rather than a global retardation of brain aging [17].

General Metabolism

Low-protein diets or caloric-restricted feeding are known to be associated with significantly reduced circulating levels of T_4 and T_3. Within 7 days of underfeeding, in rats maintained on approximately 50% ad libitum food intake, depressed levels of T_4 were apparent and were maintained until approximately 500 days of age. Returning previously dietary-restricted animals to ad libitum feeding for 7 days was sufficient to restore T_4 levels to or above normal values. Restricted feeding depressed circulating T_3 levels to a greater degree than observed for T_4 (being approximately 40% of normal values within 3–4 days of initiating restricted feeding at weaning) [1]. The intrinsic hormonal effects of T_4 are considered to contribute only a small proportion (10–15%) to the overall thyroidal status of target tissues [18], for most of the hormonal potency is derived from its conversion to T_3 at peripheral sites. During caloric restriction in the rat, the total body conversion of T_4 to T_3 is significantly reduced [19]. Thus, in this model system there is a greater peripheral effect on the conversion of T_4 to T_3, than a central neuroendocrine response to modify the release of T_4 by thyroid-stimulating hormone (TSH).

A large amount of experimental evidence indicates that the administration of T_3 stimulates RNA and protein synthesis in rat liver [20] and a direct effect of T_3 on the elongation rate of hepatic protein synthesis has been shown [21]. The depressed levels of total protein synthesis observed for liver in vivo in dietary-restricted animals [22] during the 1st year of life are associated with a significantly increased time required to assemble the average polypeptide on the ribosome. With age, however, transit time in fully fed animals increases but that of dietary-restricted animals decreases. It has been proposed that the decrease in protein synthesis observed with age in many organisms [23] results mainly from decreased rates of peptide elongation, an observation recorded in brain, kidney, liver and skeletal muscle of mice [24]. The increased ribosome transit time observed in young dietary-restricted rats was T_3-dependent, as 3 days of exogenous T_3 administration restored transit times to near normal values and increased the rate of liver protein synthesis. Refeeding previously dietary restricted rats while accelerating total protein synthesis in the liver through increased initiation sites, was not as effective as T_3 administration in restoring transit time values. A period of 28 days ad libitum feeding was required to bring the elongation time for protein synthesis to control values. A persistent, impaired T_4 to T_3 peripheral monodeiodination is present in refed dietary-restricted rats for although T_4 levels are rapidly restored to or above control values within a few days of refeeding, T_3 values remain depressed.

Chronic dietary restriction is recognized to delay the developmental decline in protein turnover in the animal as a whole, which results in significantly higher fractional synthetic rates and degradation rates for restricted animals from 1 year of age [1]. At least six hormones or groups of hormones are recognized to modify the rate of protein turnover: insulin, growth hormone (GH), somatomedins, glucagon, thyroid hormones, corticosteroids and prostaglandins. The response of some of these hormones to dietary restriction has been studied in detail [for a review, see 25]. It has been suggested that at least part of the reduction in the ability to synthesize protein with age may be due to a decline in GH secretion and, indeed, in the skeletal muscle of old ad-libitum-fed rats protein synthesis can be restored by GH administration. Conversely, the administration of *L*-dopa, a precursor of brain catecholamines, will restore GH pulse amplitude and mean GH plasma concentrations in old male rats to that observed in their young counterparts [26]. GH in young male rats is secreted in pulses every 3–4 h and this periodicity of GH release is maintained in young dietary-restricted animals. However, although the frequency of release of GH is unaffected, peak duration is reduced in such animals [25]. GH, either directly or by stimulating somatomedin-C release, increases amino acid uptake into tissues and initiates DNA transcription through the synthesis of poly-A+ RNA and the synthesis of protein [27]. To the authors' knowledge no detailed studies on the frequency of GH release in old dietary-restricted rats have been published. It may be inferred that the age-related decreased amplitude of GH pulses will be less severe in dietary-restricted rats since GH release is dependent upon the turnover of the hypothalamic catecholamines, norepinephrine and dopamine, which is preserved in these animals. Despite decreased circulating levels of GH in young underfed rats it was not possible to enhance the growth rate in these animals by exogenous administration of ovine GH. It therefore appears that such animals are not GH-deficient.

Rosenfeld et al. [28] have demonstrated a subtle synergistic induction of GH biosynthesis in the pituitary by glucocorticoids and thyroid hormones, operating through the induction of GH mRNA and thereby modifying the rate of transcription of the GH gene. While the thyroidal status of dietary-restricted animals is depressed by modification of the peripheral conversion of T_4 to T_3 (see above), the decreased release of adrenal glucocorticoids, as evident from the response of plasma corticosterone to an environmental stress, is controlled by a central neuroendocrine mechanism [25]. Circulating adrenocorticotropic hormone (ACTH) and hypothalamic releasing factors have not been measured in dietary-restricted rats. It was possible, however, to demonstrate an elevation in plasma corticosterone in response to infused ACTH in young, conscious, free-moving animals with indwelling cannulae. This observation would indicate that it is a failure to elevate plasma ACTH, rather than end-organ insensitivity induced by underfeeding, that is the cause of the lack of response to the environmental stress.

Reproductive System

In the female rat increased longevity can be achieved by chronic moderate dietary restriction, that is 50% of ad libitum food intake, without inhibition of sexual maturation or loss of fertility. Similarly, in male rats, although puberty is slightly delayed by up to 20 days, dietary-restricted animals are fertile and show a decline in fertility with age similar to their fully fed counterparts. In both sexes the most noticeable endocrine disturbance resulting from initiation of underfeeding at weaning is a premature prepubertal fall in follicle-stimulating hormone (FSH) which may be responsible for the observed delay in puberty. In the female dietary-restricted animal the prepubertal period is associated with depressed circulating progesterone values and significantly elevated circulating estradiol-17β levels [29]. As observed for the depressed corticosterone plasma values the decrease in circulating progesterone resulted from a lack of gonadotropin stimulation rather than end-organ insensitivity [25]. After sexual maturation more than 70% of dietary-restricted females demonstrated a normal 5-day estrous cycle characteristic of the strain. Chronic dietary restriction abolishes the typical age-related increase in cycle length, while delaying the appearance of the cycle irregularities so that normal estrous cycles are maintained to a much greater age in these animals. The age-related irregularities in the estrous cycles of fully fed rats have been attributed to changes in ovarian endocrine secretion and reduced capacity of the hypothalamic-pituitary system to respond to gonadal hormone feedback [30].

Detailed examination of the serum profiles for the pituitary hormones, luteinizing hormone (LH) and FSH and the ovarian steroidal hormones, progesterone and estradiol-17β in fully fed and dietary-restricted rats at 9 months of age supports the idea that retarded endocrine aging is present in the underfed animals [31]. Clear differences are present in the temporal relationship of the individual hormones between the two dietary groups, the preovulatory LH peak being reduced in height by dietary restriction and occurring approximately 6 h earlier in the cycle, whereas a delay of 6 h was observed in the rise of estradiol-17β. The total amount of estradiol-17β and progesterone released in dietary-restricted females across the cycle was reduced but there were significantly higher levels of FSH.

The retardation of the rate of endocrine aging, as reflected in the plasma levels of steroidal hormones across the 5-day cycle was confirmed in in vitro studies in which the steroidogenic pathways to estradiol-17β were examined in individual follicles [1]. With increasing age in fully fed females there was enhanced synthesis in vitro of progesterone in response to LH and increased aromatization of available androgen, resulting in a greater activity of the delta-4 pathway to estradiol-17β and decreased progesterone metabolism. These age changes were retarded by chronic dietary restriction and there was no difference in the profile of follicular steroid synthesis when follicles from 1-year-old dietary-restricted females were compared to follicles from 4-month fully fed animals. In contrast, however, follicles from 1-year-old ad-libitum-fed rats demonstrated enhanced estradiol-17β synthesis across all stages of the cycle and a significantly elevated response to LH and testosterone was recorded. Conversely, the release of testosterone and 20α-OH progesterone was reduced. Not until 600 days did follicles from underfed animals begin to show some age changes with the elevation of estradiol-17β occurring at the estrus and metestrus phases of the cycle and a concomitant decrease in the progesterone metabolic pathway.

It is not clear whether the retarded aging of the steroidogenic pathways in follicles from the ovaries of dietary-restricted rats represents an intrinsic effect of dietary restriction on the ovary, or whether it is secondary to changes in the hypothalamic-pituitary axis. Aging of the reproductive system can also be retarded by addition of *L*-tyrosine to the diet of rats from 7.5 months of age, which results in an extension of the period of estrous cyclicity. Ovariectomy of young mice followed by kidney capsule grafts of ovaries at 2 years results in retention of the capacity for cyclic LH release 6–12 months beyond the normal age and a retardation of histological changes in the arcuate nucleus, known to cause a defect in dopamine transmission in the tuberoinfundibular region, associated with high prolactin secretion and neuronal degeneration. It has been suggested [32] that cumulative steroid impact has a detrimental effect on unspecified hypothalamic and pituitary loci, resulting in a loss of neuroendocrine sensitivity to estrogen, a smaller LH surge and cycle lengthening. The lengthening of the estrous cycles is prevented by ovariectomy at a young age and some of the neuroendocrine impairments in constant-estrus animals can be reversed by prolonged ovariectomy. Finch has proposed that aging of the neuroendocrine regulating system is suspended, at least temporarily, during the period of ovariectomy by lack of steroidal action. Therefore, it can be envisaged in dietary-restricted animals that the cumulative damage to these unspecified hypothalamic and pituitary areas would occur at a slower rate because of the reduced circulating levels of steroid hormones.

Clearly, hypothalamic-pituitary aging in the dietary-restricted female rat is proceeding at a slower rate as is evident from the extension in reproductive life span in these animals. Sprague-Dawley (CFY) female rats maintained on restricted feeding from weaning at 21 days were able to produce multiple live litters as late as 937 days, an age far exceeding that recorded for animals on ad libitum feeding. Similar periods of extended reproduction have been observed in mice dietary-restricted for 6–17 months then returned to full feeding, and also in tryptophan-deficient rats returned to full feeding [1].

Immune System

The control of the immune system is predominantly genetic since the early immunological effects of underfeeding are very strain-dependent in mice. Young restricted female $B_{10}C_3F_1$ mice outperformed controls in assays of T cell function whereas the converse situation was observed in C57BL/6J mice. However, it is well established that the neuroendocrine system modulates immune function, and there is an increasing body of data which suggests that immune coordination may also be under direct neural control since electrolytic lesions in the hypothalamus induce severe involution in the thymus of the rat [33]. Conversely, the observation that immune cells secrete hormonal-like factors (including TSH, ACTH and β-endorphin) which can feed back on the neuroendocrine system suggests a complex homeostatic relationship which can clearly be modified by nutrition.

A major factor in the enhanced survival of dietary-restricted rodents is both a delay in the timing of appearance and a reduction in the incidence of many age-related pathologies, associated with a prolonged maintenance of immunological competence. Not only are dietary-restricted animals resistant to endogenous tumor formation but they also develop a degree of protection against tumor formation by exogenous carcinogens [1]. An understanding of the neuroendocrine control of the immune system under chronic dietary-restriction conditions is clearly of great importance.

In laboratory rodents thymus involution occurs shortly after puberty, an observation that has suggested that this lymphoid organ may act as a pacemaker of immunological aging [34]. In male rats, using restricted feeding and return to full feeding, it is possible to manipulate the timing of maximum size and regression in the thymus. Such a manipulation has the effect of dissociating the timing of thymus maturation from the occurrence of puberty. Surgical hypophysectomy or congenital hypopituitarism as it occurs in dwarf (dw/dw) mice results in hypotrophy of the thymus, which can be restored to normal size by administration of GH and thyroxine. The growth rate of the thymus is greatly influenced by the thyroidal status of the animal, which is chronically depressed in dietary-restricted animals [25]. In old, normal mice which have low levels of T_3 and an involuted thymus the implantation of a neonatal syngeneic thymus under the kidney capsule induces a significant increment in T_3 levels. The hormones normally considered to be involved in the modulation of the immune response are GH, TSH, ACTH, gonadotropins, thyroxine, adrenal glucocorticoids, gonadal steroids and insulin. In general, glucocorticoids, androgens, estrogens and progesterone depress the immune response in vivo, whereas GH, thyroxine and insulin increase the response. In chronic dietary-restricted animals there is a general overall reduction in circulating gonadal steroids and adrenal glucocorticoids, at least during the 1st year of life, which may be responsible in part for the enhanced immune response in these animals.

It now appears that the immune and neuroendocrine systems represent a totally integrated circuit in that components of both can produce similar peptide hormones and their receptors. The production of irACTH and endorphins by lymphocytes and Met-enkephalin by activated T helper cells suggests an immunoregulatory feedback loop that can operate by way of, or independently from, the hypothalamic-pituitary axis. Because the molecules produced by each system can feed back and regulate their own production, intrasystem feedback control is also a possibility [35]. To the authors' knowledge no data are available on the effect of chronic dietary restriction on this bidirectional neuroendocrine immunoregulation.

Discussion

The biochemical mechanism by which dietary restriction retards the rate of aging in rodents has still not been resolved. While the relationship between the antiaging actions of hypophysectomy and food restriction are unclear, a number of authors have sought to explain the mode of action of restricted feeding through a modification of the neuroendocrine system. It is clear that the early idea of dietary-induced pseudohypophysectomy leading to prolonged periods in an arrested prepubertal state reflected merely the severity of the early restricted feeding regimes and is not a necessary prerequisite for extended longevity. The work of Segall et al. [9] using diets low in tryptophan together with the work of Fernstrom and Wurtman [10], has raised the possibility that the concentrations of particular essential amino acids can modify neurotransmitter synthesis, thereby providing a direct link between the environment and neuroendocrine function. The suggestion that the neuroendocrine axis is central to the mode of action of dietary restriction provides a physiological system through which gene expression and ontogenetic processes are modified and metabolic homeostasis is maintained. The recently established bidirectional interplay of the immune and neuroendocrine systems provides the theoretical basis whereby the retention of immunocompetence and the delay in the expression of many pathologies of aging in these animals can be accommodated.

Although basic data on the endocrine response to dietary restriction have been published, much of the detail regarding the control of gene expression or the regulation of immune function remains to be determined in these animals. While it is, therefore, plausible to construct hypotheses regarding the mechanisms of action of dietary restriction based on complex neuroendocrine adjustments, such ideas do not identify the basic molecular changes occurring in individual cells in response to restricted feeding. Specifically, in tryptophan-deficient diets the amino acid is equally important in regulating polysome profiles, and in the thyroidal response to underfeeding the major effect appears to be related to the peripheral conversion of T_4 to T_3 rather than major changes in central neuroendocrine control. Whether the decrement in peripheral monodeiodination of T_4 to T_3 is the response to further endocrine changes within the animal is unknown.

In rodents with delayed aging induced by controlled underfeeding enhanced protein turnover at advanced chronological age has been demonstrated for the whole animal, and for particular tissues in vivo and in vitro. It can be argued that the retention of a higher rate of protein turnover to advanced age protects against the accumulation of labile or damaged proteins and provides a fine degree of metabolic control for proteins with a regulatory role. Whether the neuroendocrine system plays a major role in determining the rate of protein turnover in these animals is unknown but the endocrine control of protein synthesis may be the molecular expression of the neuroendocrine system to dietary restriction.

References

1 Holehan, A.M.; Merry, B.J.: The experimental manipulation of ageing by diet. Biol. Rev. *61:* 329–368 (1986).
2 Segall, P.E.: Interrelations of dietary and hormonal effects in aging. Mech. Age. Dev. *9:* 515–525 (1979).
3 McCay, C.M.; Maynard, L.A.; Sperling, G.; Barnes, L.L.: Retarded growth, lifespan, ultimate body size and age changes in the albino rat after feeding diets restricted in calories. J. Nutr. *18:* 1–13 (1939).
4 Meites, J.; Goya, R.; Takahashi, S.: Review article. Why the neuroendocrine system is important in aging processes. Exp. Gerontol. *22:* 1–15 (1987).
5 Everitt, A.V.; Seedsman, N.J.; Jones, F.: The effects of hypophysectomy and continuous food restriction, begun at ages 70 and 400 days, on collagen aging, proteinuria, incidence of pathology and longevity in the male rat. Mech. Age. Dev. *12:* 161–172 (1980).
6 Everitt, A.V.; Porter, B.: Nutrition and aging; in Everitt, Burgess, Hypothalamus, pituitary and aging, pp. 570–613 (Thomas, Springfield 1976).

7 Campbell, G.A.; Kurcz, M.; Marshall, S.; Meites, J.: Effects of starvation in rats on serum levels of follicle stimulating hormone, thyrotropin, growth hormone and prolactin: response to LH releasing hormone and thyrotropin releasing hormone. Endocrinology *100:* 580–587 (1977).

8 Harrison, D.E.; Archer, J.R.; Astle, C.M.: The effect of hypophysectomy on thymic aging in mice. J. Immun. *129:* 2673–2677 (1982).

9 Segall, P.E.; Timiras, P.S.; Walton, J.R.: Low tryptophan diets delay reproductive aging. Mech. Age. Dev. *23:* 245–252 (1983).

10 Fernstrom, J.D.; Wurtman, R.J.: Effect of chronic corn consumption on serotonin content of rat brain. Nature *234:* 62–64 (1971).

11 Munro, H.N.; Hubert, C.; Baliga, B.S.: Regulation of protein synthesis in relation to amino acid supply – a review; in Rothschild, Oratz, Schreiber, Alcohol and abnormal protein synthesis, biochemical and clinical, pp. 33–66 (Pergamon, New York 1975).

12 Enesco, H.E.; Kruk, P.: Dietary restriction reduces fluorescent age pigment accumulation in mice. Exp. Gerontol. *16:* 357–361 (1981).

13 Walker, R.F.; McMahon, K.M.; Pivorun, E.B.: Pineal gland structure and respiration as affected by age and hypocaloric diet. Exp. Gerontol. *13:* 91–99 (1978).

14 Levin, P.; Haji, M.; Joseph, J.A.; Roth, G.S.: Effect of aging on prolactin regulation of rat striatal dopamine receptor concentrations. Life Sci. *32:* 1743–1749 (1983).

15 Joseph, J.A.; Whitaker, J.; Roth, G.S.; Ingram, D.K.: Life-long dietary restriction affects striatally-mediated behavioral responses in aged rats. Neurobiol. Aging *4:* 191–196 (1983).

16 Roth, G.S.; Ingram, D.K.; Joseph, J.A.: Delayed loss of striatal dopamine receptors during aging of dietarily restricted rats. Brain Res. *300:* 27–32 (1984).

17 London, E.D.; Waller, S.B.; Ellis, A.T.; Ingram, D.K.: Effects of intermittent feeding on neurochemical markers in ageing rat brain. Neurobiol. Aging *6:* 199–204 (1985).

18 Oppenheimer, J.H.; Dillman, W.H.: Nuclear receptors for triiodothyronine: a physiological perspective; in Birnbaumer, O'Malley, Receptors and hormone action, pp. 1–33 (Academic Press, New York 1978).

19 Van Doorn, J.; Van Der Heide, D.; Roelfsema, F.: The influence of partial food deprivation on the quantity and source of triiodothyronine in several tissues of athyreotic thyroxine-maintained rats. Endocrinology *115:* 705–711 (1984).

20 Bernal, J.; Coleoni, A.H.; De Groot, L.J.: Triiodothyronine stimulation of nuclear protein synthesis. Endocrinology *102:* 452–459 (1978).

21 Mathews, R.W.; Oronsky, A.; Haschemeyer, A.E.V.: Effect of thyroid hormone on polypeptide chain assembly kinetics in liver protein synthesis in vivo. J. biol. Chem. *248:* 1329–1333 (1973).

22 Merry, B.J.; Holehan, A.M.; Lewis, S.E.M.; Goldspink, D.F.: The effects of ageing and chronic dietary restriction on in vivo hepatic protein synthesis in the rat. Mech. Age. Dev. *39:* 189–199 (1987).

23 Makrides, S.C.: Protein synthesis and degradation during aging and senescence. Biol. Rev. *58:* 343–422 (1983).

24 Blazejowski, C.A.; Webster, G.C.: Effect of age on peptide chain initiation and elongation in preparations from brain, liver, kidney and skeletal muscle of the C_{57}BL/6J mouse. Mech. Age. Dev. *25:* 323–333 (1984).

25 Merry, B.J.; Holehan, A.M.: The endocrine response to dietary restriction in the rat; in Woodhead, Blackett, Hollaender, The molecular biology of aging. Basic Life Scis, vol. 35, pp. 117–141 (Plenum, New York 1985).
26 Sonntag, W.E.; Hylka, V.W.; Meites, J.: Growth hormone restores protein synthesis in skeletal muscle of old male rats. J. Geront. *40:* 689–694 (1985).
27 Knobil, E.; Hotchkiss, J.: Growth hormone. A. Rev. Physiol. *26:* 47–74 (1964).
28 Rosenfeld, M.G.; Amara, S.G.; Birnberg, N.C.; Mermod, J.-J.; Murdoch, G.H.; Evans, R.M.: Calcitonin, prolactin and growth hormone gene expression as model systems for the characterization of neuroendocrine regulation. Recent. Prog. Horm. Res. *39:* 305–351 (1983).
29 Holehan, A.M.; Merry, B.J.: The control of puberty in the dietary restricted female rat. Mech. Age. Dev. *322:* 179–191 (1985).
30 Lu, J.K.H.: Changes in ovarian function and gonadotropin and prolactin secretion in aging female rats; in Meites, Neuroendocrinology of aging; pp. 103–122 (Plenum, New York 1983).
31 Holehan, A.M.; Merry, B.J.: Modification of the oestrous cycle hormonal profile by dietary restriction. Mech. Age. Dev. *32:* 63–76 (1985).
32 Finch, C.E.; Felicio, L.S.; Mobbs, C.; Nelson, J.F.: Ovarian and steroidal influences on neuroendocrine aging processes in female rodents. Endocr. Rev. *5:* 467–497 (1984).
33 Isakovic, K.; Jankovic, M.T.: Neuro-endocrine correlates of immune response. II. Changes in the lymphatic organs of brain-lesioned rats. Int. Archs Allergy *45:* 373–384 (1973).
34 Kay, M.M.B.: The thymus: clock for immunologic aging? J. invest. Derm. *73:* 29–38 (1979).
35 Blalock, J.E.; McMenamin, D.H.; Smith, E.M.: Peptide hormones shared by the neuroendocrine and immunologic systems. J. Immun. *135:* 858s–861s (1985).

Dr. B.J. Merry, Wolfson Institute, University of Hull, Hull HU6 7RX (UK)

Interdiscipl. Topics Geront., vol. 24, pp. 74–80 (Karger, Basel 1988)

Adrenocortical Cell Turnover and Aging in Growth-Retarded Rats

(With 1 color plate)

Judie Walton[a], *James Pruss*[a], *Arthur V. Everitt*[b,1]

[a]CSIRO Prospect, Australia; [b]Department of Geriatric Medicine, University of Sydney, Repatriation General Hospital, Concord, Australia

Introduction

There are several ways to retard aging, delay age-related pathology, and prolong the life of the laboratory rat. This can be achieved by dietary restriction of total calories, of protein, or of an essential amino acid such as tryptophan. Hypophysectomy has a similar action. At the present time, the exact mechanism(s) by which these treatments retard aging is unknown. In order to understand why tissue structure and functions such as hormone synthesis change with age, we are examining how age-retarding treatments alter cell turnover rates and tissue composition. The adrenal cortex is particularly appropriate for this type of study because its cells are arranged in an orderly sequence according to their maturity.

Age Change and Cell Turnover in Adrenal Cortex

The adrenal cortex is comprised of three morphologically distinct areas. The zona glomerulosa is outermost and its stem cells divide to give rise to newly differentiated adrenal cells. Over the next few months, the

[1] The authors wish to thank the Gerontology Foundation of Australia and the National Health and Medical Research Council (grant No. 865073) for contributing toward the cost of this publication.

adrenocyte is displaced inwardly [1], producing a gradient of younger to older cells from the zona glomerulosa, to the zona fasciculata, and finally to the zona reticularis which surrounds the adrenal medulla. When young, the adrenocyte synthesizes aldosterone; upon leaving the zona glomerulosa it produces glucocorticoids, and upon reaching the zona reticularis it produces sex hormones [1].

In the guinea pig adrenal cortex, mitotic rates decrease with age [2]. There is evidence that the zona glomerulosa of rat atrophies with time [3], and in our study the mitotic index (percent dividing cells in the zona glomerulosa) decreased from 0.08% in the young rat (3 months) to 0.04% by middle age (13 months). Adrenocortical cell division in the oldest group (30–34 months) was close to zero. It was too low to obtain a reliable quantitation by mitotic count and would require a more sensitive technique such as autoradiography.

Age pigment is a well-known marker of old cells. In the adrenal cortex of young rats, this fluorescent pigment was only seen in a few degenerating cells in a region, bordering the medulla, which corresponds to the zona reticularis of older animals.

In middle-aged and old control rats, this zone contained considerable numbers of the pigment-laden cells which are probably degenerating as part of the normal cell turnover process.

Age pigment has been found throughout the adrenal cortex of naturally aged, senescent rats, particularly within the zona reticularis [4]. Our results agree with this and we were impressed by the large numbers of zona glomerulosa cells containing pigment granules in the oldest group. We interpreted this to indicate that many cells within this compartment were not being displaced to the zona reticularis within 120 days as reported for adrenocytes from young rats [1]. In middle-aged controls, pigment was not conspicuous in the zona glomerulosa but small granules were found in adrenocytes throughout the zona reticularis and in deeper regions of the zona fasciculata.

Diminution in rates of protein synthesis [5], with ribosome loss [6], is a well-established feature of older tissues so that protein content can be used as a rough guide to cell age. In comparison to tissue from young rats, adrenocortical tissue from old rats took up less eosin which stains protein.

At the ultrastructural level, adrenocytes from our old animals showed less cytoplasmic flocculent material which is generally considered to represent protein.

Age Change and Cell Turnover in Adrenal Cortex of Growth-Retarded Rats

In growth-retarded rats, morphological age changes occur more slowly so adrenocortical cells of old food-restricted rats more closely resembled cells from healthy, middle-aged controls. Compared to age-matched controls, cells from old (30–34 months) food-restricted rats took up more eosin stain and, in electron micrographs, they showed more flocculent material in their cytoplasm, indicating a higher protein content.

Age pigment in the old food-restricted rat adrenal was primarily confined to the zona reticularis. As in middle-aged controls, there were some pigment-containing cells in the zona fasciculata and none were seen in the zona glomerulosa. Old food-restricted rats not only had fewer pigmented cells but the granules were also smaller and more sparsely distributed than in cells of old controls (fig. 1, 2).

Mitotic rates in the food-restricted animals did not show such a steep decline with time as in controls and thus allowed cell turnover to continue at a relatively constant level into old age. The mitotic index was 0.04% for adrenal stem cells from old food-restricted rats, being more similar to the middle-aged controls than to their age-matched counterparts which had too few mitoses to be counted.

The higher mitotic rates, smaller amounts of age pigment, and greater protein content of food-restricted rats all indicate that their adrenal cells were, on the average, chronologically younger than comparable cells in age-matched controls; that is they were generated from mitoses more recently.

Mitotic figures were not seen in old hypophysectomized adrenal cortex but a complicating factor in identifying metaphase plates in these cells was that they had highly irregular nuclear profiles. Very little age pigment was visible in any adrenocortical zone of the old hypophysectomized rats and only small numbers of degenerating cells could be seen near the medulla. In these ways the old hypophysectomized tissue resembled the adrenal cortex of young control animals.

Adrenal glands of old hypophysectomized animals were very small and their cells were probably relatively inactive, considering that their metabolism is normally adrenocorticotropic-hormone-dependent. The indications of slower turnover in these cells (low mitosis, few degenerating cells) suggests that they are aging more slowly than adrenocytes of control animals and that age pigment accumulation is probably related to cell metabolic activity.

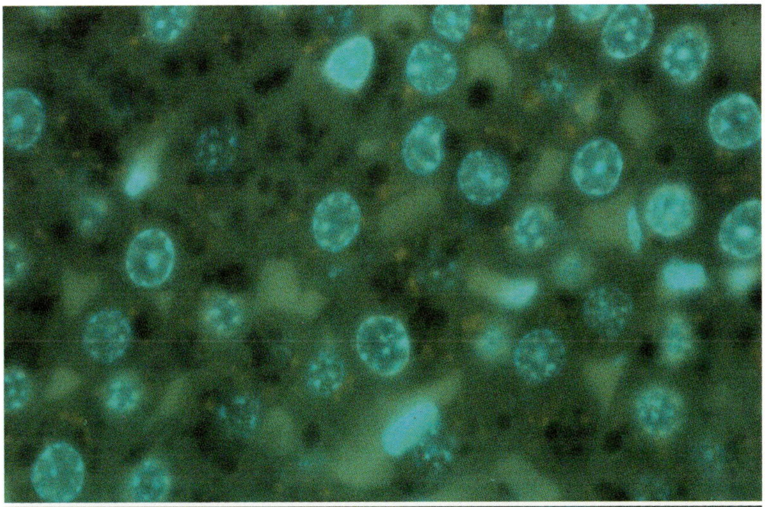

1

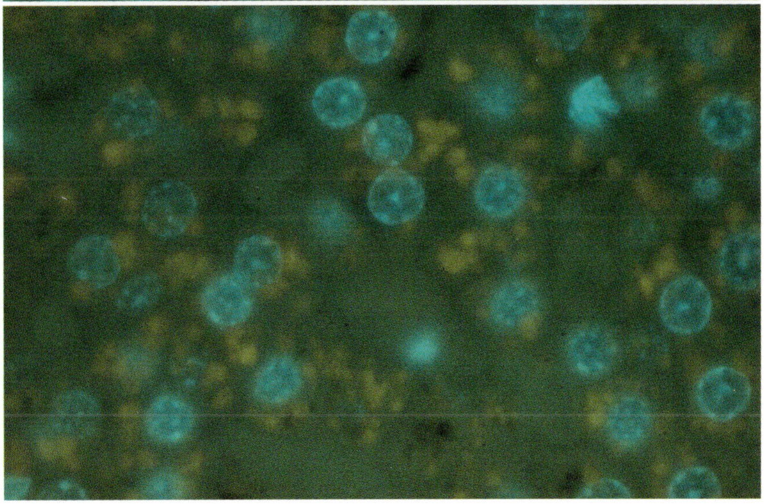

2

Fig. 1, 2. Zona reticularis cells from old rats (approximately 33 months). DNA in nuclei fluoresce blue and age pigment granules yellow. *1* Adrenocortical cells from an old food-restricted rat. *2* Adrenocortical cells from an old control rat. Note that the granules are larger and more numerous than in cells of the old food-restricted animal.

Cell Division, Usage, and Aging

Each type of differentiated cell has a limited functional life. For some, this time is measurable in years (e.g. neurons) but other types of cells survive for only days (e.g. gingival and gastrointestinal lining cells). The turnover time for rat adrenocytes is intermediate, averaging about 120 days [1]. In general, to maintain optimum function – even in young tissue – old defunct cells need to be regularly replaced by new ones arising from stem cell mitoses.

Within an animal's life span, differentiated cells can be used either for (1) embryogenesis, (2) body growth, or (3) tissue repair and maintenance. During the first two phases more cells are being produced than are being spent so the body grows. In the third phase, cell production is in balance with cell depletion so tissue structure and function are effectively maintained.

In most tissues, mitotic rates fall throughout life and when cell production no longer keeps pace with cell loss, tissue renewal is impaired and aging becomes evident. The tissue begins to show atrophy, which manifests either quantitatively as cell deficit or qualitatively as structural deterioration with progressive rise in the average age of the cell population. Both conditions are accompanied by functional involution.

There is considerable evidence in the gerontological literature that the age-related mitotic decline shown by all kinds of somatic stem cells is due to intrinsic, genetically determined limits on their ability to divide [for a review, see 7]. The rates at which cells divide are regulated by hormones, growth factors, mitogens, and chalones. High levels of many hormones and nutrients increase mitotic rates so that more stem cells reach their genetically determined limit earlier. Conversely, food restriction and hypophysectomy, by reducing nutrient supply and hormone secretion, curb cell division and so delay the rate at which cells approach their genetic limits. This, evidently, is the reason that adrenals of old food-restricted and hypophysectomized rats have mitotic indices similar to those of middle-aged controls.

While hormones and other circulating substances can accelerate and slow cell mitotic rates, there has been no evidence that they can reinitiate division in a cell line which has exhausted its replication potential. For example, hormones do not stimulate the production of new neurons or oocytes in human adults.

Most, if not all, tissues show some amount of mitotic decline within the life span. Presumably, the net falloff in mitotic indices reflects the decreasing balance of stem cells which still have division potential as one by one they lose this capacity. Declining mitotic rates limit the total numbers of differentiated cells produced in that tissue within the individual's life span. Both food restriction and hypophysectomy, by slowing this decline, allow a more continuous supply of newly differentiated cells to be produced.

Body Size and Longevity

It has long been recognized that body size and longevity are related. The nature of this correlation depends on genetic relationship. For mammals of different species, large animals tend to live longer than smaller species. Also, cells from larger, longer-lived animals have a greater capacity for cell division in vitro when compared to the same type of cells from smaller, shorter-lived species [8]. Size, longevity, and in vitro mitotic activity are all expressions of a species' cell replication potential.

Within a single species, paradoxically, smaller animals generally tend to live longer than larger ones. For example, small dogs can survive up to 25 years whereas very large dogs seldom live beyond 10–12 years although both types are descendants of a medium-sized ancestor and their genomes are similar enough to allow matings. Also, within a species, mammalian females tend to be smaller than males with significantly longer life spans. The implication is that cell usage can be genetically redirected from growth into longevity increase. Virtually the same intraspecies effect is seen in hypophysectomized or nutritionally restricted animals where longevity increase is greatest when growth is least.

Age-retarding treatments all stunt growth by inhibiting protein synthesis [9], which in turn retards cell division. In these animals, the adrenals and most other organs are proportionate to body size and therefore smaller than in control animals and they do not show pathological age change until considerably later ages.

Altered Cell Usage and Life Prolongation

Everitt [10] and others have shown that old hypophysectomized and food-restricted rats not only live longer but the tensile strength of their tail collagen fibers resembles that of young control animals, they have low tumor incidence, and they show less pathological change characteristic of the aging process. How can these observations be explained in the present context?

Firstly, in hypophysectomized and nutritionally restricted animals, the inhibitory effects on protein synthesis would also reduce the activity of cross-linking enzymes. Hence, fibers would be less cross-linked and more similar to those of younger animals.

Secondly, there is the observation of very low tumor incidence. The relationship between cancer and aging is not yet clear but Ponten [11] has noted that rare childhood cancers generally develop in tissues at a time when cell divisions are drastically slowing. Thus, neuroblastomas occur around the time the brain has reached full size and osteoblastomas develop soon after skeletal growth subsides. This implies that as stem cells near their final divisions, they are much more prone to mutation or nondisjunction. If this concept holds for other age-related tumors, hypophysectomized and food-restricted animals may not develop tumors at normal rates of incidence because their cell replicative capacity in the various tissues is not as close to depletion as in the age-matched controls.

Finally, how could the delay in onset of age-related pathologies be explained? Experimental treatments are usually begun at 1 month of age or just after weaning. By this time embryogenesis is well over but body growth is incomplete. If cell divisions are allowed to proceed normally, the animal grows to its full size and begins to show muscle wastage and other evidence of tissue deterioration on schedule. We hypothesize that in animals on these growth-restricting, life-prolonging regimens, some mitoses which would normally contribute to growth to produce a larger body are instead diverted into tissue renewal and repair. Because this allows a cell supply adequate to offset cell attrition, the smaller adrenals and other organs are kept in a younger, more healthy condition until a later age, giving the growth-retarded rat an extended life span.

References

1 Zajicek, B.; Ariel, I.; Arber, N.: The streaming adrenal cortex: direct evidence of centripetal migration of adrenocytes by estimation of cell turnover rate. J. Endocr. *111:* 477–482 (1986).

2 Blumenthal, H.T.: The mitotic count in the adrenal cortex of normal guinea pigs. Growth *27:* 477–480 (1940).

3 Dunihue, F.W.: Reduced juxtaglomerular cell granularity, pituitary neurosecretory material, and width of the zona glomerulosa in aging rats. Endocrinology *77:* 948 (1965).
4 Reichel, W.: Lipofuscin pigment accumulation and distribution in five rat organs as a function of age. J. Geront. *23:* 145–153 (1968).
5 Makrides, S.C.: Protein synthesis and degradation during aging and senescence. Biol. Rev. *58:* 343–422 (1983).
6 Miquel, J.; Johnson, J.E., Jr.: Senescent changes in the ribosomes of animal cells in vivo and in vitro. Mech. Age. Dev. *9:* 247–266 (1979).
7 Walton, J.R.: The role of limited cell replicative capacity in pathological age change. A review. Mech. Age. Dev. *19:* 217–244 (1982).
8 Rohme, D.: Evidence for a relationship between longevity of mammalian species and life spans of normal fibroblasts in vitro and erythrocytes in vivo. Proc. natn. Acad. Sci. USA *78:* 5009–5013 (1981).
9 Holehan, A.M.; Merry, B.J.: The experimental manipulation of ageing by diet. Biol. Rev. *61:* 329–368 (1986).
10 Everitt, A.V.: Hypophysectomy and aging in the rat; in Everitt, Burgess, Hypothalamus, pituitary and aging, pp. 68–85 (Thomas, Springfield 1976).
11 Ponten, J.: Abnormal cell growth (neoplasia) and aging; in Finch, Hayflick, Handbook of the biology of aging, pp. 536–560 (Van Nostrand & Reinhold, New York 1977).

Dr. Judie Walton, CSIRO, PO Box 239, Blacktown, NSW 2148 (Australia)

Interdiscipl. Topics Geront., vol. 24, pp. 81–89 (Karger, Basel 1988)

Neuroendocrine System, Programmed Cell Death, and Aging

Rodolfo G. Goya

Endocrine Studies Center/Oncological Center for Excellence,
National University of La Plata / J.M. Mainetti Foundation, La Plata, Argentina

The occurrence of cell death as a programmed phenomenon is a well-established fact in developmental biology. Programmed cell death is a regular event during morphogenesis and the means whereby embryonal and larval organs are eliminated [1, 2]. Programmed cell death also plays a relevant role in plant physiology in general [3] and in the senescence and death of monocarpic (annual) plants, in particular [4]. So far, however, programmed cell death has aroused very little interest among gerontologists.

The main purpose of the present chapter is to call the reader's attention to this unexplored avenue of gerontological research. In doing so, the first part will be devoted to describing the basic features of programmed cell death. Next, the hormonal control of senescence and cell death in plants will be briefly reviewed. In the two following sections the experimental evidence pointing to the neuroendocrine system as the potential regulator of cell death during aging will be discussed. Since the idea of cell death during aging being under neuroendocrine control is univocally linked to the hypothesis that senescence is a programmed event, the last section will be devoted to discussing the viability of this hypothesis.

Characteristics of Physiological Cell Death

Although the hypotheses underlying the concepts of physiological cell death and programmed cell death are not the same, for all practical purposes these terms can be considered equivalent. Therefore, programmed cell death and physiological cell death will be used interchangeably throughout this chapter.

Almost all cells undergoing physiological death follow an orderly and characteristic sequence of structural changes called apoptosis [5, 6]. These changes take place in two discrete stages. The first involves nuclear and cytoplasmic condensation, and breaking up of the cell into a number of membrane-bound, ultrastructurally well-preserved fragments. In the second stage these apoptotic bodies are shed from epithelial-lined surfaces or are taken up by other cells – where they undergo a series of changes resembling in vitro autolysis within phagosomes – and are rapidly degraded by lysosomal enzymes derived from the ingesting cell.

The fact that cells undergoing apoptosis within tissues are usually surrounded and outnumbered by viable cells has made it difficult to obtain biochemical information about physiological cell death. Nevertheless, there are a few cell systems where apoptosis can be initiated synchronously and in enough numbers of cells to allow biochemical studies. Regressing mammary tumors are perhaps the best characterized models [7]. Physiological cell death seems to be an energy-dependent process which requires synthesis of RNA and protein at least during its early stages [8, 9].

Apoptosis appears to play a complementary role to mitosis in regulating the dynamics of cell populations. Its morphological and biochemical features suggest that it is an inherently programmed phenomenon that can be initiated or inhibited by a variety of extracellular stimuli, both physiological and pathological [10].

Physiological cell death is a cell-limited process where inflammation or contamination of the intercellular milieu by lysosomal enzymes does not occur [11]. Furthermore, apoptosis markedly differs from coagulative necrosis which classically results from injury by agents such as toxins or ischemia, and involves massive cell death accompanied by exudative inflammation [8, 12].

It has been hypothesized that the capability of cells for self-destruction arose at the early stages of evolution of multicellular eukaryotes, conferring them the ability to readily eliminate nonfunctional or harmful cells and, later in evolution, becoming the basis for the appearance of complex morphogenetic processes [13]. Whether there is any relationship between physiological cell death and in vitro cell aging and death [14] remains to be elucidated.

Programmed Cell Death during Senescence in Plants

Plants are the only organisms where programmed cell death has a fairly well-established role during senescence. Furthermore, senescence itself is a programmed event in plants. Hence, it is of interest to discuss briefly the subject here. In plant physiology, the terms senescence and aging have clearly different meanings. Senescence is an active degenerative process leading to death and is internally controlled. Aging is a passive process caused more directly by external factors as time passes [15]. Senescence is intimately associated with many phases of plant development. Most studies on plant senescence have focused on particular organs rather than processes; leaves have been most extensively studied, followed by flowers and fruits [16–18]. Nevertheless, interest in whole plant senescence has increased in recent years and so has the understanding of its complex control mechanisms [4]. Cell death during plant senescence appears as an orderly process where ribosomes and chloroplasts show the first symptoms of deterioration, while mitochondria and nuclei change later, and the cell and vacuolar membranes last of all [19]. Senescence in plants involves synthesis of new proteins and is an energy-dependent process [20]. Degradation is a common feature of senescent plant cells and has the important function of releasing and redistributing the nutrients invested in the senescing tissues.

Plant senescence and cell death seem to be predominantly under hormonal control. Very often a specific cell or an organ is induced to senesce by signals from other parts of the plant. These signals are called correlative controls and coordinate the activities of different parts of the plant or tissue [21].

There are two general categories of plant hormones involved in control of senescence. The senescence-retarding hormones like cytokinins, auxins, and gibberellins seem to prevent or delay the initiation of senescence in leaves and petals [19]. Cytokinins are mainly synthesized by the root tips of the plant, and the decline in the cytokinin levels reaching the leaves is part of the signal that triggers foliar senescence [4, 22]. The senescence-promoting hormones represent the second group of messengers. They include ethylene, which appears to be the primary inducer of flower senescence [17], and abscisic acid involved mainly in foliar senescence [23]. In monocarpic plants (like soybean) senescence and death of the whole plant is a clearly programmed event [4]. The senescence signal for the whole plant comes from the developing fruit but its identity remains unknown [24].

Neuroendocrine Control of Cell Death during Development

Perhaps the best known instance of programmed cell death controlled by the neuroendocrine system is the sequence of cataclysmic phenomena during amphibian metamorphosis in which thyroid hormones initiate the degeneration of the intestinal epithelium and several tissues of the tail [25]. In insects, ecdysis (shedding of the hard exoskeleton) is often followed by programmed cell death in some structures which are no longer useful. In many cases this process has been shown to be under neuroendocrine control. Thus, in silkmoths, the postecdysial degeneration of the abdominal intersegmental muscles is triggered by eclosion hormone, a peptide released by the insect's nervous system at the time of eclosion [26, 27]. The postecdysial degeneration of the wing epidermis in blowflies is initiated by another neurohormone, bursicon [28, 29]. Among other invertebrates, a cerebral neurosecretion in the mollusc Crepidula controls the regression of the muscle fibers of the penis at the time of sexual inversion [30].

Deleterious Consequences of Neuroendocrine Function after Puberty

In mammals, puberty is the last event where the involvement of a developmental program is still evident. Puberty may be regarded as a triggering event which begins the gradual decline in homeostatic potential that characterizes aging. Of particular significance is the fact that thymus involution begins after puberty. This early involution has led many to regard the thymus gland as the pacemaker of immunological aging [31]. Furthermore, the increasing evidence that the immune and neuroendocrine systems function as a bidirectional network suggests that the deleterious consequences of thymic involution may extend beyond the immune system itself [32, 33].

Thymus regression involves both cell emigration [34] and cell death in situ [35], the latter having the features of apoptosis [36]. There is compelling evidence suggesting that thymic involution, like puberty, is triggered by the neuroendocrine system: adrenal and sexual steroids have a powerful inhibitory effect on thymocytes [36, 37]. Furthermore, adrenalectomy or castration are followed by hypertrophy of the thymus [38]. Interestingly, castration in old male rats is followed by a spectacular recovery of thymic mass and morphology, indicating that even the low levels of circulating testosterone in the old males are exerting a significant inhibitory action on the thymus [39]. Grafting of GH_3 pituitary cells, which secrete prolactin and growth hormone, was also able to restore thymus size and function in old rats [40]. Plasma growth hormone is known to decline with age in rats [41, 42].

A different line of evidence also points to a deleterious action of the hypophysis during aging. In 1974, Denckla [43] reported the partial purification of a pituitary factor that decreased the reponse of peripheral tissues to thyroid hormone with age. Although no further characterization of this factor has been reported, this author and others have observed a restorative effect of long-term hypophysectomy on the decline of many functions with age. Thus, it has been shown that long-term hypophysectomy, followed by minimal hormone replacement therapy, delays the decrease of minimal oxygen consumption in old rats [43], restores the ability to reject xenografts and clear carbon in middle-aged rats [44], prevents the age-associated decrease in RNA synthesis initiation in rat liver [45], and partially prevents the decline in some immunological activities with increasing age [46].

Hypophysectomy in rats also delays collagen aging and the age-associated increase of protein excretion in urine [47], as well as the hind limb paralysis and gastrocnemius muscle degeneration typically observed in very old animals [48].

Programmed Aging as a Viable Possibility

There is general agreement that, up to puberty, the different stages an organism goes through are genetically programmed. There are two basic possibilities after sexual maturity is reached: (a) both the reproductive period and the aging process are genetically programmed, or (b) the developmental program runs out at some point after sexual maturation takes place. In this case, the length of the reproductive period would be determined by the degree of perfection of the homeostatic systems of the adult organism. Senescence would appear when these systems begin to run over tolerance. Although both hypotheses remain viable so far, the involvement of programmed cell death in the aging process can be discussed only within the framework of the first hypothesis, namely that aging is a programmed phenomenon. The possibility that aging is a programmed process under neuroendocrine control has been previously suggested [49–52].

An argument frequently raised against the idea of programmed senescence is that there is no *obvious* selective advantage in keeping a genetic program for a postreproductive event. While the argument is theoretically solid from an evolutionary point of view, the evidence that monocarpic plants do undergo programmed senescence has the strength of the experimental facts. It may well be that programmed senescence evolved only in some species, perhaps those with fewer natural predators.

It has been suggested that turnover is a basic feature of living systems, ranging from biomolecules to ecosystems [15]. Within this attractive hypothesis it is intellectually effortless to view physiological cell death and programmed senescence as the respective counterparts to mitosis and reproduction.

Conclusion

Programmed cell death may hold fundamental clues for the understanding of the aging process, and research efforts in this area may prove unsuspectedly rewarding.

One of the fundamental questions in basic gerontology is whether or not senescence is a programmed step of life. If future research established a relevant role for programmed cell death during aging, and this process were demonstrated to be under the control of the neuroendocrine system, then the hypothesis of senescence in higher organisms being the last part of a general developmental program controlled by the neuroendocrine system would become strongly supported.

Acknowledgements

The author is a recipient of an NIH Biomedical Support Grant from the College of Veterinary Medicine, Michigan State University. The author is grateful to Dr. Joseph Meites, Dr. Richard Lockshin, and Dr. Larry Noodén for their helpful comments, to Ms. Yolanda Sosa for assistance in the bibliographic search, and to Dr. Victoria Kingsbury for editorial assistance and typing of the manuscript.

References

1 Hinchliffe, J.R.: Cell death in embryogenesis; in Bowen, Lockshin, Cell death in biology and pathology, p. 35 (Chapman & Hall, New York 1981).
2 Lockshin, R.A.: Cell death in metamorphosis; in Bowen, Lockshin, Cell death in biology and pathology, p. 79 (Chapman & Hall, New York 1981).

3 Barlow, P.W.: Cell death – an integral part of plant development; in Jackson, Grout, Mackenzie, Growth regulators in plant senescence, monograph 8, p. 27 (British Plant Growth Regulator Group, Wantage 1982).
4 Noodén, L.D.: Senescence in the whole plant; in Thimann, Senescence in plants, p. 219 (CRC Press, Boca Raton 1980).
5 Kerr, J.F.R.; Wyllie, A.H.; Currie, A.R.: Apoptosis: a basic biological phenomenon with wide-ranging implications in tissue kinetics. Br. J. Cancer *26:* 239–257 (1972).
6 Wyllie, A.H.; Kerr, J.F.R.; Currie, A.R.: Cell death: the significance of apoptosis. Int. Rev. Cytol. *68:* 251–306 (1980).
7 Gullino, P.M.: Mechanism of regression in hormone-dependent mammary carcinomas; in McGuire, Breast cancer, vol. 3, p. 51 (Plenum, New York 1979).
8 Wyllie, A.H.: Cell death: a new classification separating apoptosis from necrosis; in Bowen, Lockshin, Cell death in biology and pathology, p. 9 (Chapman & Hall, New York 1981).
9 Lockshin, R.A.: Nucleic acids in cell death; in Davies, Sigee, Cell ageing and cell death, p. 243 (Cambridge University Press, Cambridge 1984).
10 Kerr, J.F.R.: Shrinkage necrosis: a distinct mode of cellular death. J. Pathol. *105:* 13–20 (1971).
11 Gullino, P.M.; Lanzerotti, R.H.: Mammary tumor regression. II. Autophagy of neoplastic cells. J. natn. Cancer Inst. *49:* 1349–1356 (1972).
12 Judah, J.D.; Ahmed, K.; McLean, A.E.M.: Pathogenesis of cell necrosis. Fed. Proc. *24:* 1217–1221 (1965).
13 Umansky, S.R.: The genetic program of cell death. Hypothesis and some applications: transformation, carcinogenesis, ageing. J. theor. Biol. *97:* 591–602 (1982).
14 Hayflick, L.: Cell death in vitro; in Bowen, Lockshin, Cell death in biology and pathology, p. 243 (Chapman & Hall, New York 1981).
15 Leopold, C.A.: Aging and senescence in plant development; in Thimann, Senescence in plants, p. 1 (CRC Press, Boca Raton 1980).
16 Thimann, K.V.: The senescence of leaves; in Thimann, Senescence in plants, p. 85 (CRC Press, Boca Raton 1980).
17 Mayak, S.; Halevy, A.H.: Flower senescence, in Thimann, Senescence in plants, p. 131 (CRC Press, Boca Raton 1980).
18 Rhodes, M.J.C.: The maturation and ripening of fruits; in Thimann, Senescence in plants, p. 157 (CRC Press, Boca Raton 1980).
19 Noodén, L.D.; Thompson, J.E.: Aging and senescence in plants; in Finch, Schneider, Handbook of the biology of aging; 2nd ed., p. 105 (Van Nostrand & Reinhold, New York 1985).
20 Noodén, L.D.; Leopold, A.C.: Phytohormones and the endogenous regulation of senescence and abscission; in Letham, Goodwin, Higgins, Phytohormones and related compounds – a comprehensive treatise, vol. 2, p. 329 (Elsevier/North Holland Biomedical Press, Amsterdam 1978).
21 Leopold, A.C.; Noodén, L.D.: Hormonal regulatory systems in plants; in Scott, Encyclopedia of plant physiology, vol. 10, p. 4 (Springer, New York 1984).
22 Kende, H.: The cytokinins. Int. Rev. Cytol. *31:* 301–338 (1971).
23 Sacher, J.A.: Abscisic acid in leaf senescence; in Addicott, Abscisic acid, p. 479 (Praeger, New York 1983).

24 Noodén, L.D.: Integration of soybean pod development and monocarpic senescence. A minireview. Physiol. Plant. *62:* 273–284 (1984).
25 Dodd, M.J.H.; Dodd, J.M.: The biology of metamorphosis; in Lofts, Physiology of the amphibian, vol. 3, p. 467 (Academic Press, New York 1976).
26 Schwartz, L.M.; Truman, J.W.: Peptide and steroid regulation of muscle degeneration in an insect. Science *215:* 1420–1421 (1982).
27 Truman, J.W.; Schwartz, L.M.: Peptide hormone regulation of programmed death of neurons and muscle in an insect; in Bloom, Peptides, integrators of cell and tissue function, vol. 35, p. 55 (Raven Press, New York 1980).
28 Reynolds, S.E.: Bursicon; in Downer, Laufer, Invertebrate endocrinology, vol. 1: Endocrinology of insects, p. 235 (Liss, New York 1983).
29 Seligman, I.M.; Doy, F.A.: Hormonal regulation of disaggregation of cellular fragments in the haemolymph of *Lucilia cuprina.* J. Insect Physiol. *19:* 125–135 (1973).
30 Streiff, W.; Le Gall, S.: Etude ultrastructurale de la dégénérescence des myocytes du pénis sous l'influence du facteur dédifférenciateur cérébral chez *Crepidula fornicata* (phil.) (mollusque hermaphrodite protrandre). Colloques int. Cent. natn. Rech. scient. *251:* 139–147 (1976).
31 Kay, M.M.B.: The thymus: clock for immunologic aging? J. invest. Derm. *73:* 29–38 (1979).
32 Fabris, N.; Piantanelli, L.: Thymus-neuroendocrine interactions during development and aging; in Adelman, Roth, Endocrine and neuroendocrine mechanisms of aging, p. 167 (CRC Press, Boca Raton 1982).
33 Meites, J.; Goya, R.; Takahashi, S.: Why the neuroendocrine system is important in aging processes. Exp. Gerontol. *22:* 1–15 (1987).
34 Sainte-Marie, G.; Peng, F.S.: Emigration of thymocytes from the thymus. A review and study of the problem. Revue can. Biol. *30:* 51–78 (1971).
35 Hinsull, S.M.; Bellamy, D.; Franklin, A.: A quantitative histological assessment of cellular death, in relation to mitosis, in rat thymus during growth and age involution. Age Ageing *6:* 77–84 (1977).
36 La Pushin, R.W.; Harven, E.: A study of gluco-corticosteroid-induced pyknosis in the thymus and lymph node of the adrenalectomized rat. J. Cell Biol. *50:* 583–597 (1971).
37 Grossman, C.J.: Interactions between the gonadal hormones and the immune system. Science *227:* 257–261 (1985).
38 Comsa, J.: Hormonal interactions of the thymus; in Luckey, Thymic hormones, p. 59 (University Park Press, Baltimore 1973).
39 Greenstein, B.D.; Fitzpatrick, F.T.A.; Adcock, I.M.; Kendall, M.D.; Wheeler, M.J.: Reappearance of the thymus in old rats after orchidectomy: inhibition of regeneration by testosterone. J. Endocr. *110:* 417–422 (1986).
40 Kelley, K.W.; Brief, S.; Westly, H.J.; Novakofski, J.; Bechtel, P.J.; Simon, J.; Walker, E.B.: GH_3 pituitary adenoma cells can reverse thymic aging in rats. Proc. natn. Acad. Sci. *83:* 5663–5667 (1986).
41 Sonntag, W.E.; Steger, R:W.; Forman, L.J.; Meites, J.: Decreased pulsatile release of growth hormone in old male rats. Endocrinology *107:* 1875–1879 (1980).
42 Takahashi, S.; Gottschall, P.E.; Quigley, K.L.; Goya, R.G.; Meites, J.: Growth hormone secretory patterns in young, middle-aged and old female rats. Neuroendocrinology *46:* 137–142 (1987).

43 Denckla, W.D.: Role of the pituitary and thyroid glands in the decline of minimal O_2 consumption with age. J. clin. Invest. *53:* 572–581 (1974).
44 Bilder, G.E.; Denckla, W.D.: Restoration of ability to reject xenografts and clear carbon after hypophysectomy in adult rats. Mech. Age. Dev. *6:* 153–163 (1977).
45 Miller, J.K.; Bolla, R.; Denckla, W.D.: Age-associated changes in initiation of ribonucleic acid synthesis in isolated rat liver nuclei. Biochem. J. *188:* 55–60 (1980).
46 Scott, M.; Bolla, R.; Denckla, W.D.: Age related changes in immune function of rats and the effect of long-term hypophysectomy. Mech. Age. Dev. *11:* 127–136 (1979).
47 Everitt, A.V.; Wyndham, J.R.; Barnard, D.L.: The anti-aging action of hypophysectomy in hypothalamic obese rats: effects on collagen aging, age-associated proteinuria development and renal histopathology. Mech. Age. Dev. *22:* 233–251 (1983).
48 Everitt, A.V.; Shorey, C.D.; Ficarra, M.A.: Skeletal muscle aging in the hind limb of the old male Wistar rat: inhibitory effect of hypophysectomy and food restriction. Archs Gerontol. Geriatr. *4:* 101–115 (1985).
49 Finch, C.E.: The regulation of physiological changes during mammalian aging. Q. Rev. Biol. *51:* 49–83 (1976).
50 Denckla, W.D.: A time to die. Life Sci. *16:* 31–44 (1975).
51 Everitt, A.V.: The genetic clock-hormone theory of aging; in Biological and social aspects of mortality and the length of life, p. 279 (Ordina, Liège. 1982).
52 Goya, R.G.: Role of programmed cell death in the aging process: an unexplored possibility. Gerontology *32:* 37–42 (1986).

Dr. Rodolfo Goya, Centro de Estudios Endócrinos,
Facultad de Medicina, U.N.L.P., Casilla de correo 455, La Plata 1900 (Argentina)

Interdiscipl. Topics Geront., vol. 24, pp. 90–97 (Karger, Basel 1988)

Regulation of Age-Related Changes in Hypothalamo-Pituitary-Ovarian Function in the Mouse

Lêda S. Felicio [a, d], *James F. Nelson* [b–d]

Departments of [a] Medicine and [b] Obstetrics and Gynecology,
[c] Center for Studies in Age and Aging, [d] Center for the Study of Reproduction,
McGill University, Royal Victoria Hospital, Montreal, Que., Canada

Introduction

Although many aspects of reproductive aging are widely shared among strains and species, there is a considerable heterogeneity in the timing of these changes as well as in their regulation [18, 19, 21]. As a consequence, caution must be taken when extrapolating results from one species or strain to another, and it is important to distinguish between events and mechanisms of reproductive aging which are common across species and those which have a more limited distribution. This chapter reviews knowledge on the regulation of reproductive aging in one rodent strain, the inbred C57BL/6J mouse, with the caveats noted above. Previous reviews provide comparisons of this model with others [18, 19].

Use of the phrase, 'regulation of female reproductive aging', is not meant to imply that the decline in reproductive function is a genetically programed process similar to those occurring during development. It is more likely that reproductive aging, as all aging processes, is the consequence of the *reduced* selection pressures that inevitably occur with advancing chronological age [23, 24]. The term 'regulation' is used to emphasize that the *mechanisms* leading to and underlying reproductive failure are the primary focus of this chapter – not the age-related changes themselves. Detailed descriptions of these changes – the loss of ovulatory cyclicity and fertility and their hormonal correlates – are well documented

[7, 18, 19], and therefore will only be briefly reviewed. The C57BL/6J mouse strain is emphasized because there is little data available on other strains. Thus, the generality of the observations, even for *Mus musculus*, remains to be determined.

Age-Related Changes in Estrous Cyclicity

Increases in the length of the estrous cycle and its variability are among the earliest changes during reproductive aging. Around 9–10 months of age, the modal cycle length increases from 4–5 days, and, in those animals that continue to cycle, the average cycle length, as well as its variability, continues to increase [16, 17]. Pseudopregnant-like periods also occur during the transition to acyclicity, but these are rare [8]. Cessation of cyclicity occurs between 10 and 14 months of age, and is often followed by a period of persistent vaginal cornification [4]. The incidence of persistent vaginal cornification as well as its duration are inversely proportional to the age of onset of acyclicity [4]. Persistent vaginal cornification is followed by a state of persistent diestrus, which continues until death.

Endocrine Correlates of Reproductive Aging

Age-related changes in the serum profiles of estradiol (E_2), progesterone (P_4) and luteinizing hormone (LH) occur concomitantly with the onset of cycle lengthening. The preovulatory surge of LH on the evening of proestrus in middle-aged mice is delayed and truncated, resulting in 40% reduction in integrated exposure of target tissues to elevated LH [8]. The preovulatory P_4 surge shows an even greater reduction [8]. E_2 levels are also altered at this age. Baseline levels of E_2 during the cycle are reduced and the preovulatory increase of E_2, which is the trigger for the preovulatory surge of LH, is delayed by about 1 day [16].

In acyclic mice with persistent vaginal cornification, the ovary continues to secrete sufficient estrogen to produce a cornified vaginal epithelium [4] and maintain normal baseline serum concentrations of LH [9]. Estradiol levels are low but higher than ovariectomized values [3]. This contrasts with the persistent diestrus state, which is characterized by elevated LH levels [9]. Although ovarian steroids have not been measured in mice with persistent diestrus, the hypergonadotropic condition associated with this state [9] along with the atrophic condition of the vagina and uterus indicate that ovarian secretory activity is minimal.

Regulation of Reproductive Aging

Both the Ovary and the Neuroendocrine System Play a Role

The physiological events of reproductive aging are thus well documented, as are many of the corresponding hormonal and, to a lesser extent, biochemical changes [7, 18, 19, 21, 22]. The question that remains largely unanswered is: what regulates these changes? Specifically, what controls the lengthening of cycles and their ultimate termination? Are the changes in hormonal profiles causal or merely correlative? If causal, what in turn is responsible for their alteration? Answering these questions involves searching for the acute regulatory factors as well as the initiating causes – factors that may have long-term cumulative effects.

To answer these questions, our strategy has been to identify the components of the hypothalamo-pituitary-ovarian axis that contribute to a given change in reproductive function during aging, and then to begin to dissect those components to find the mechanisms responsible for their contribution. To distinguish ovarian causes from extraovarian causes (the latter will hereafter be presumed to be neuroendocrine in origin) we have employed a procedure introduced by Krohn [13] as a tool for understanding aging processes: heterochronic tissue transplantation. Using this approach, he replaced ovaries of middle-aged CBA mice with ovaries from young donors and thereby restored the cyclicity of the hosts [14]. This was the first study to show conclusively that ovarian aging was the principle component regulating the cycling life span of a species. Age changes extrinsic to the ovary (i.e. neuroendocrine) were secondary insofar as this aspect of reproductive failure was concerned.

Our studies using heterochronic ovarian grafting have revealed that the relative importance of the aging ovary and the neuroendocrine system varies with each event of reproductive aging. Thus, cessation of cyclicity is primarily due to ovarian failure, whereas cycle lengthening has both neuroendocrine and ovarian causes [6]. This is demonstrated by the observation that young ovaries grafted into mice about to cease cycling extend the cycling life span of those mice by about 60%. This result shows that the potential of the neuroendocrine system to sustain cyclicity extends well beyond that of the ovary. Despite a lengthened period of cyclicity, the cycle lengths of middle-aged mice bearing young ovaries are not restored to the modal 4-day status of young mice [6]. The incidence of longer cycles (i.e. cycles > 5 days) is reduced, however, in these middle-aged hosts of young ovaries. Our interpretation of these results is that neuroendocrine changes play the major role in the early increase from 4- to 5-day cycles, whereas there is an important ovarian contribution to the increase in cycles longer than 5 days in middle-aged mice.

Ovarian Changes

What, then, are the changes in ovarian and neuroendocrine function that underlie their respective contributions to cycle lengthening and cessation? With respect to the ovary, changes in the number and function of ovarian follicles are likely to play a major role. The follicle, which encircles the oocyte, is the source of the hormonal secretions that trigger the hypothalamo-pituitary unit to release the gonadotropic signal which induces ovulation and thereby maintains cyclicity. Thus, declining follicular reserves or alterations in the remaining follicles are likely candidates for the ovarian contribution to cessation of cyclicity and cycle prolongation [18, 19]. Little is known about the functional integrity of the remaining follicles in the aging ovary, but the effects of aging on the numbers of follicles and the role of their decline have been studied. Follicle reserves decline steadily with advancing age and thus clearly set a limit to the reproductive life span of female mammals [7, 18, 19]. In rats, neuroendocrine changes occur well before follicular reserves are depleted and appear to play the major role in limiting the cycling life span [18, 22]. By contrast, the ovarian reserves appear to set the limit on cyclicity in mice [6, 14] as well as humans [20]. Follicle reserves in middle-aged C57BL/6J mice that were still cycling were twice those of age-matched mice that were anovulatory [11]. More conclusive evidence of the importance of ovarian and presumably follicular failure in the loss of cyclicity in mice was the observation discussed earlier that young ovarian grafts extended the cycling life span of middle-aged mice by about 60% [6].

Neuroendocrine Changes

In middle-aged mice, neuroendocrine changes are only sufficient to influence cycle length; they are insufficient to terminate cyclicity [6]. However, neuroendocrine dysfunction is progressive with advancing age; in 17-month-old mice, young ovaries only modestly improve cyclicity relative to untreated controls, and by 24 months grafts of young ovaries are incapable of restoring cyclicity [5], indicating that neuroendocrine failure is complete by this age.

Little is known about the neuronal changes responsible for neuroendocrine failure in mice. The ability of E_2 to induce a preovulatory-like LH surge declines with advancing age in parallel with the decline in neuroendocrine regulation of ovulation as indicated from ovarian grafting studies [7]. Thus, disruption must occur in one or more of the neuronal pathways or pituitary loci that mediate the estrogen stimulation of LH release. In females rats, altered monoamine function has been correlated with failure to elicit an LH surge [18, 19, 22] and may therefore play a role in mice, but this has not been examined. There appears to be no deficit in the number of gonadotropin-releasing-hormone-containing cells in the hypothalamus or preoptic area of middle-aged female C57BL/6J mice [12]. Thus, the failure most probably lies in the mechanisms that regulate the release of gonadotropin-releasing hormone into the portal circulation. Limited studies indicate that the pituitary responsiveness to gonadotropin-releasing hormone in terms of LH release is not altered during aging [21].

The first step in the transduction of the estrogen signal often involves the intracellular binding of estrogen to its receptor, which permits the receptor to alter gene expression and thereby elicit the changes in protein synthesis which are required for the cellular response. Recent studies indicate that the magnitude and duration of nuclear binding of the estrogen receptor following exposure to an elevated level of circulating estrogen is reduced 25–35% in the middle-aged hypothalamus [2, 15]. This alteration may contribute to the impaired responsiveness of the hypothalamus to E_2. Further studies are needed to establish whether there are additional impairments downstream from the receptor, for example in estrogen receptor gene expression, that are independent of reduced hormone receptor binding and hence may amplify the effects of reduced hormone receptor binding. In this context, it is important to recognize that small impairments in many steps of the pathway leading to hormone action may lead to an amplification of the overall impairment.

Role of Chronic Exposure to Ovarian Hormones

One of the only clues to the etiology of the decline in LH surge potential is that long-term withdrawal from ovarian secretions delays its onset [5, 7, 18, 19]. Conversely, exposure of intact or ovariectomized mice to exogenous estrogen can advance the loss of the LH surge potential [7, 18].

This suggests that chronic exposure to endogenous ovarian secretions is an etiological agent in the age-related loss of hypothalamo-pituitary function. Little is known about the mechanisms or neuroanatomical substrates that are influenced by and hence may mediate the effects of long-term ovarian steroidal exposure. However, recent studies indicate that the potentiating effects of hormonal exposure on age-related changes are selective in both the events that they influence and the periods of the life span during which they are most deleterious [19]. In addition, it is now apparent that effects of chronic estrogen exposure occur in the uterus [10] and vagina [1] as well as in the hypothalamus and pituitary.

If long-term ovariectomy is restricted to the period of regular cyclicity, it does not delay the loss of cycling potential of a middle-aged mouse, as measured by the effect of grafted young ovaries on the cycling life span [6]. By contrast, if the period of ovariectomy is extended to include several months of the postcyclic period, the cycling potential is significantly extended [5]. These and other data [19] suggest that there are periods of the life span when hormonal secretions are more deleterious, either because their patterns differ or because their targets are more vulnerable.

Conclusions

The age-related decline in the regulation of hypothalamic-pituitary-ovarian function in the mouse is a multifactorial process involving changes in both neuroendocrine and ovarian loci. Ovarian hormones play a role in these changes, both in terms of the immediate effects of altered patterns on function as well as the delayed effects of long-term exposure on target tissue responsiveness. Progress has been made in elucidating the relative contributions of the neuroendocrine and ovarian loci, as well as of hormonal exposure, to the altered function of the aging female reproductive system. Further work is needed to identify more precisely the anatomical lesions and the windows of vulnerability to hormonal exposure and the mechanisms whereby steroids potentiate reproductive aging changes.

References

1 Adler, A.J.; Nelson, J.F.: Aging and chronic estradiol exposure impair estradiol-induced cornification but not proliferation of vaginal epithelium in C57BL/6J mice. Biol. Reprod. *38:* 175–182 (1988).

2 Bergman, M.; Karelus, K.; Nelson, J.: Altered estrogen receptor dynamics in middle-aged C57BL/6J mice. Gerontologist *27:* 146A (1987).

3 Felicio, L.S.; Nelson, J.F.; Finch, C.E.: Spontaneous pituitary tumorigenesis and plasma oestradiol in ageing female C57BL/6J mice. Exp. Gerontol. *15:* 139–143 (1980).

4 Felicio, L.S.; Nelson, J.F.; Finch, C.E.: Longitudinal studies of estrous cyclicity in aging C57BL/6J mice. II. Cessation of cyclicity and the duration of persistent vaginal cornification. Biol. Reprod. *31:* 446–453 (1984).

5 Felicio, L.S.; Nelson, J.F.; Gosden, R.G.; Finch, C.E.: Restoration of ovulatory cycles by young ovarian grafts in aging mice: potentiation by long-term ovariectomy decreases with age. Proc. natn. Acad. Sci. USA *80:* 6076–6080 (1983).

6 Felicio, L.S.; Nelson, J.F.; Finch, C.E.; with the technical assistance of Jacobson, B., and McLean, M.: Prolongation and cessation of estrous cycles in aging C57BL/6J mice are differentially regulated events. Biol. Reprod. *34:* 849–858 (1986).

7 Finch, C.E.; Felicio, L.S.; Mobbs, C.V.; Nelson, J.F.: Ovarian and steroidal influences on neuroendocrine aging processes in female rodents. Endocr. Rev. *5:* 467–497 (1984).

8 Flurkey, K.; Gee, D.M.; Sinha, Y.N.; Finch, C.E.: Age effects on luteinizing hormone, progesterone, and prolactin in proestrus and acyclic C57BL/6J mice. Biol. Reprod. *26:* 835–846 (1982).

9 Gee, D.M.; Flurkey, K.; Finch, C.E.: Aging and the regulation of luteinizing hormone in C57BL/6J mice: impaired elevations after ovariectomy and spontaneous elevations at advanced ages. Biol. Reprod. *28:* 598–607 (1983).

10 Goodrick, G.; Nelson, J.: The effect of food restriction and long-term ovariectomy on the decidual cell response in aging mice. Gerontologist *27:* 146A (1987).

11 Gosden, R.G.; Laing, S.C.; Felicio, L.S.; Nelson, J.F.; Finch, C.E.: Imminent oocyte exhaustion and reduced follicular recruitment mark the transition to acyclicity in aging C57BL/6J mice. Biol. Reprod. *28:* 255–260 (1983).

12 Hoffman, G.E.; Finch, C.E.: LHRH neurons in the female C57BL/6J mouse brain during reproductive aging: no loss up to middle age. Neurobiol. Aging *7:* 45–48 (1986).

13 Krohn, P.L.: Review lectures on senescence. II. Heterochronic transplantation in the study of aging. Proc. R. Soc. *157:* 128–147 (1962).

14 Krohn, P.L.: Transplantation and aging; in Krohn, Topics in the biology of ageing, pp. 125–148 (Wiley, New York 1966).

15 Nelson, J.F.; Bergman, M.; Karelus, K.; Felicio, L.S.: Aging of the hypothalamo-pituitary-ovarian axis: hormonal influences and cellular mechanism. J. Steroid Biochem. *27:* 699–705 (1987).

16 Nelson, J.F.; Felicio, L.S.; Osterburg, H.H.; Finch, C.E.: Altered profiles of estradiol and progesterone associated with prolonged estrous cycles and persistent vaginal cornification in aging C57BL/6J mice. Biol. Reprod. *24:* 784–794 (1981).

17 Nelson, J.F.; Felicio, L.S.; Randall, P.K.; Simms, C.; Finch, C.E.: A longitudinal study of estrous cyclicity in C57BL/6J mice. I. Cycle frequency, length and vaginal cytology. Biol. Reprod. *27:* 327–339 (1982).

18 Nelson, J.F.; Felicio, L.S.: Reproductive aging in the female: an etiological perspective. Rev. biol. Res. Aging *2:* 251–314 (1985).

19 Nelson, J.F.; Felicio, L.S.: Reproductive aging in the female: an etiological perspective updated. Rev. biol. Res. Aging *3:* 359–381 (1987).

20 Richardson, S.J.; Senikas, V.; Nelson, J.F.: Follicular depletion during the menopausal transition: evidence for accelerated loss and ultimate exhaustion. J. clin. Endocr. Metab. *65:* 1231–1237 (1987).

21 Vom Saal, F.S.; Finch, C.E.: Reproductive: senescence. phenomena and mechanisms in mammals and selected vertebrates; in Knobil, Pfaff, Greenwald, Physiology of reproduction, pp. 2351–2413 (Raven Press, New York 1987).

22 Wise, P.M.: Aging of the female reproductive system. Rev. biol. Res. Aging *1:* 195–222 (1983).

23 Williams, G.C.: Pleiotropy, natural selection, and the evolution of senescence. Evolution *11:* 398–411 (1957).

24 Williams, G.C.: Adaptation and natural selection (Princeton University Press, Princeton 1966).

Dr. James Nelson, Obstetrics and Gynecology, McGill University,
Royal Victoria Hospital, Women's Pavilion, 687 Pine Avenue West,
Montreal, PQ, H3A 1A1 (Canada)

Interdiscipl. Topics Geront., vol. 24, pp. 98–110 (Karger, Basel 1988)

Glucocorticoid Receptors, Stress and Aging

Ramesh Sharma[1], *Paola S. Timiras*

Department of Physiology-Anatomy, University of California, Berkeley, Calif., USA

Overview

What are the causes of the decreased ability to respond to stress in old age? One among many hypotheses focuses on the hypothalamopituitary-adrenal axis as a key regulator of homeostasis and adaptation; however, other organs, such as the lungs, kidneys, liver and gut are also involved. Maintenance of homeostasis involves a complex series of integrative functions in which almost all body organs and systems participate, albeit in varying degrees. Thus, homeostatic competence provides a 'panoramic view' of overall physiological performance and explains the current interest among physiologists to identify the control mechanisms involved in this integrated activity.

Under resting (basal) conditions few changes occur in hypothalamopituitary-adrenal function with increasing age. Similarly, fasting blood sugar levels remain constant throughout the life span and the blood acidity and bicarbonate content are closely regulated, even into advanced age. In contrast, the rate at which the body is able to readjust and return to normal resting values after the experimental alteration of blood sugar, bicarbonate, or a stress situation stimulating adrenal response is much slower in old subjects than in young. As functional performance declines with increasing age and as pathological events accumulate and become more severe, the capacity of the organism to synchronize defensive and homeostatic mechanisms is concomitantly impaired. Thus, the failure of the elderly to adapt

[1] Ramesh Sharma offers thanks to the Ministry of Human Resources and Development, Government of India for the National Scholarship and the University of Manipur for the study leave.

to internal and external environmental changes reflects more the inability to purposefully coordinate several functions involved in supporting homeostasis than the failure of any single function (although the failure of one may provide a trigger) [1, 2].

Evidence of decreased resistance to environmental changes accompanying the aging process is plentiful and the increased risk of death following stress in the elderly is acknowledged. Older people are less resistant than younger subjects to excessively cold or warm temperatures due to the progressive deterioration of thermoregulatory mechanisms. Equally diminished is the capacity to adapt to hypoxia, traumatic injury, exercise, and physical work, all types of stress that require complex physiological adjustments. For example, the ability to carry out physical work involves competence of numerous functions, such as oxygen uptake by the lungs and/or tissues, pulmonary ventilation, diffusing capacity of lungs, cardiac work, pulse rate, and production and elimination of blood lactate. Alteration in any of these factors or their interrelation will result in a marked decrease in work capacity and a significant increase in the time for recovery from exercise. Emotional stress in the old may also trigger or aggravate a series of physical ailments that, superimposed on an already debilitated state, would lead to disease and death.

Some of the aging changes of the adrenal cortex and medulla and those in the nervous system may be responsible for the decline in adaptive capability. Stressful stimuli activate both the hypothalamopituitary-adrenocortical and sympathoadrenal systems which coordinate physiological reactions to maintain homeostasis. This coordination is through a series of neuroendocrine signals which involve various hormones and brain centers. Aging disrupts the synchrony of these signals: the capacity to restore the original homeostasis is altered and the hypothalamus is unable to undergo the major remodeling of its circuitry necessary for adaptation [3].

The role of the hypothalamopituitary-adrenal system in adaptive responses was first emphasized by Cannon [4] for the adrenal medulla and by Selye and Prioreschi [5] for the adrenal cortex. This role has been both supported and criticized by many investigators and continues to be controversial. However, only recently have advances in neuroendocrinologic knowledge and techniques established more solid cellular and molecular bases for these views. For example, at the cellular level, abnormalities of protein metabolism with stress have been implicated as contributing to the degenerative changes leading to the pathology of dementias; at the molecular level, loss of glucocorticoid receptors in selected brain neurons may release the hypothalamopituitary-adrenocortical system from the inhibitory action of limbic structures with consequent failure to adapt [6]. We shall be considering in this review the relationship between glucocorticoid receptors, stress and aging.

Glucocorticoid Receptors – Regional Distribution and Characteristics

Glucocorticoids such as cortisol and corticosterone have a multitude of effects within the body. They generate appropriate physiological (metabolic) adjustments necessary for the responses to stress [7]. The major effects of glucocorticoids, in response to stress and environmental insults, are to reduce inflammation, stabilize blood glucose, maintain muscle strength, and promote fluid excretion. These hormones are secreted from the adrenal cortices under the control of the brain via pituitary, hypothalamus and limbic system. Various environmental and psychological stimuli activate the release of corticotropin-releasing hormone (CRH) from the hypothalamus, CRH in turn stimulates the pituitary adrenocorticotropic hormone (ACTH) which regulates the secretion of glucocorticoids from the adrenal gland [8]. Glucocorticoids are involved in defense mechanisms to stress, both at central and peripheral levels. These effects, turning on and off of the adrenal-pituitary axis are mediated through pituitary, hypothalamus and limbic brain regions (fig. 1).

The glucocorticoid receptors are located in most target tissues. High-affinity glucocorticoid receptors have been demonstrated in different brain regions [9–11]. The highest concentrations of glucocorticoid receptors are present in the hippocampus (fig. 2). Due to the presence of high level of glucocorticoid receptors, the hippocampus is believed to be a mediator of glucocorticoid effects on the brain. It is referred to as a 'window' through which glucocorticoids modulate such complex activities of central nervous system (CNS) as mood, motivation and learned behaviors [12]. The presence of glucocorticoid receptors in CNS supports the role of glucocorticoids in switching on and off the stress responses through negative feedback [13]. Glucocorticoid effects on the brain are highly diversified: they influence monoamines, neuropeptides and amino acid transmitters at the molecular level, induce cell loss at the cellular level, increase excitability and altered behavior at the functional level. These functional, cellular and molecular changes occur throughout development, adulthood and aging of organisms.

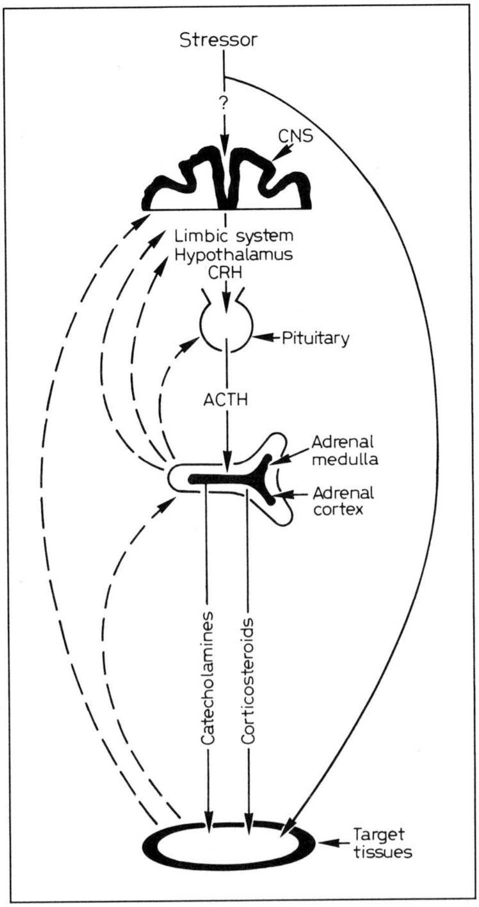

Fig. 1. Schematic representation of the postulated mechanisms of stressors on target tissues. Stressors act on the higher central nervous system (CNS) centers through mechanisms still unknown (?). Stressors may also act directly on the target tissues. Stimulation of CNS centers is relayed to the limbic system, particularly the hippocampus and from there to the hypothalamus. In the hypothalamus, synthesis and release of CRH are increased and the hormone through the portal system stimulates the anterior pituitary to increase ACTH production. ACTH, in turn, stimulates the adrenal cortex to produce more corticosteroids, which then act on target tissues. Simultaneously with the activation of the hypothalamopituitary-adrenal axis, there is also a sympathetic activation of catecholamine release from the adrenal medulla. The overall responsiveness of this complex neuroendocrine system to stressors also depends on the presence of negative feedbacks (---). Such feedbacks exist between steroid-pituitary, steroid-hypothalamus and steroid-limbic systems. The responses of target tissues may also be modulated by negative feedbacks either directly on the adrenal or CNS.

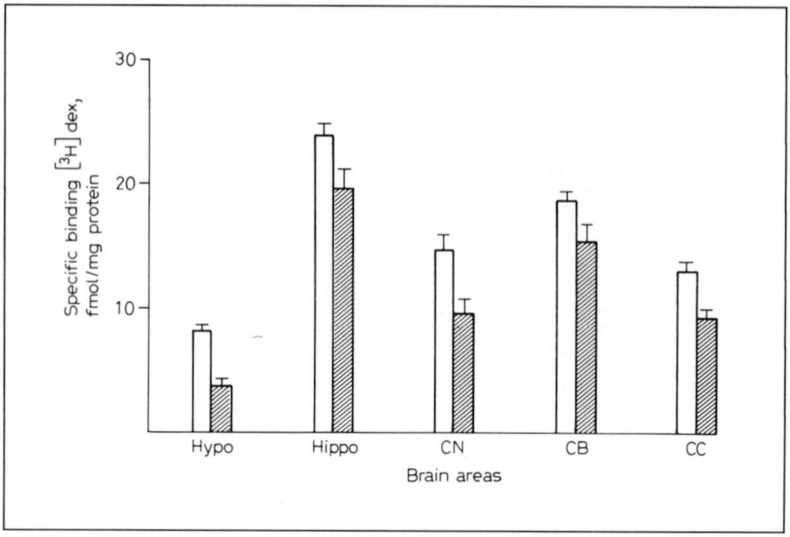

Fig. 2. Saturable cytosolic-specific binding of [^{3}H]dexamethasone ([^{3}H]dex) in hypothalamus (Hypo), hippocampus (Hippo), caudate nucleus (CN), cerebellum (CB) and cerebral cortex (CC) of 3- (□) and 26-week-old (▨) adrenalectomized Long-Evans male rats. Results are mean ± SD of the 4–5 samples collected from 4–5 rats of each age group. Note that at both ages the number of binding sites is highest in the hippocampus. The binding sites decrease with age (20–30%) in all the brain areas [38].

In vitro binding studies have revealed at least two classes of corticosteroid receptors: type 1 (mineralocorticoids) and type 2 (glucocorticoids). They differ in affinity (K_d) and specificity for certain synthetic and naturally occurring corticosteroids [10]. The physical characteristics of neural glucocorticoid receptors have been examined in several studies. Using [^{3}H]dexamethasone, a synthetic glucocorticoid, as a ligand, most investigators have reported equilibrium dissociation constant (K_d) of 2–10 n*M* [14–16] and sedimentation coefficient of 6–8 S depending on the experimental conditions [14, 15]. Isoelectric focusing studies have demonstrated the existence of a single class of dexamethasone receptors with a pI of 6.1 [15, 16]. Brain glucocorticoid receptors display most of the kinetic properties similar to those of the receptors present in other tissues such as liver, kidney and thymus [11]. These intracellular receptors upon binding to hormones are activated prior to binding to nuclear acceptor sites. The activation of steroid-receptor complexes has been described as a not well-defined, conformational change which enables the complexes to interact with specific acceptor sites on chromatin and modulate gene expression [17]. This nuclear binding capacity can be achieved in vitro by incubating the hormone-receptor complexes at 25 °C [18, 19] and under high ionic conditions [20]. Such phenomena are achieved possibly by exposure of positively changed amino acid residues on the surface of the receptor molecule, which in turn enhances the affinity for nuclei and polyanions such as DNA and DNA-cellulose [21]. The activation of glucocorticoid receptors occurs in vivo under physiological conditions and is thought to be rate-limiting for nuclear binding [22, 23].

Changes in Glucocorticoid Receptors during Development: Correlations with Adaptive Responsiveness to Stress

Adaptive responses to hormones are age-related phenomena as are changes in induction of many enzymes [24]. These hormone-mediated responses are controlled by binding of the hormone to specific intracellular receptors, by activation of hormone receptor complexes and interaction of these complexes to nuclear acceptor sites. Many of these events are altered with age [25, 26]. In the rat brain, glucocorticoid receptors are detectable as early as the 17th day of gestation. After birth, the receptor binding capacity gradually increases to adult levels by 15–30 days of age [27–29]; it also undergoes changes in physicochemical properties [26, 30, 31], which may account, at least in part, for changes with age in tissue responsiveness to glucocorticoids [32]. For example, nuclear transfer of bound hormone receptor complexes reaches mature levels only after the postnatal day 10 in the pituitary of rats. The reduced transfer of hormone receptor complexes to nuclei is correlated with the nonresponsive period to stress in neonatal rats [33]. We have observed a reduced heat activation of [^{3}H]-dexamethasone receptor complexes in the cerebral hemispheres of adult rats as compared to weanling rats [34].

The postnatal rise in the brain glucocorticoid receptors of rats during the 2nd week of life has been correlated with a low adrenocortical response to stress [35]. This period of adrenocortical unresponsiveness has been termed a 'stress-nonresponsive period'. The neonatal rats are less sensitive not only to the stimulatory effects of stress, but also to the inhibitory effects of circulating corticosterone. Administration of dexamethasone does not suppress circulating corticosterone titers in neonates, while it does in adult rats [35]. In adult animals both corticosterone and dexamethasone inhibit subsequent adrenocortical secretion. The stress nonresponsive period has shown adaptive value on the development of central nervous system since high or low levels of corticosteroids are associated with abnormal neural and behavioral growth. The neonatal adrenocortical activity corresponds to the unique pattern of glucocorticoid receptor concentrations that exist in the brain and pituitary at these phases of the life span: this low, stable corticoid level appears suitable for neuronal development in glucocorticoid-sensitive brain regions [35].

Changes in Glucocorticoid Receptors during Aging: Correlations with Adaptive Responsiveness to Stress

Glucocorticoid binding sites have been reported to decline in the cerebral hemispheres of aged (24 months) rats [36], and in isolated neuronal perikarya from the cerebral cortex of aged Sprague-Dawley rats as compared to young rats [37]. [^{3}H]dexamethasone binding sites decrease by 20–30% in different brain regions of adult male Long-Evans rats as compared to weanling rats (fig. 2) [38]. In contrast, in C57/6J mice, the corticosterone binding sites in the cytosol of hypothalamus, hippocampus or cortex remain unchanged with senescence [39]. Likewise, the number of glucocorticoid binding sites was low in the hippocampus but not in other cortical brain regions of older rats [40]. A site-specific decrease in corticosterone binding was observed in the brain of aged rats [41]. In these studies, age-dependent decrease in receptors were marked in the hippocampus and amygdala but not in the hypothalamus, cortex and midbrain. These authors further established that the reduction in hippocampal receptors was due to decreased number of corticosterone-concentrating neurons as determined by autoradiography [42]. Glial and other cell uptake of [^{3}H]-dexamethasone was not depressed in aging hippocampus [41]. The loss of hippocampal glucocorticoid receptors has been well correlated with the loss of hippocampal neuronal population in discrete subfields of Ammon's horn as a function of age [6]. These neuronal losses in aged animals have been associated with the increased glucocorticoids with age as demonstrated first in the hippocampus of guinea pigs [43]. Daily subcutaneous injection of corticosterone over 3 months led to loss of [^{3}H]dexamethasone receptor binding sites in vitro and neuronal loss in specific areas of Ammon's horn [6]. The regulation of brain corticosteroid receptors during aging seems to be a multifactorial process. The levels of glucocorticoid binding sites in neural tissues are controlled by several factors in addition to age. These factors include neural innervation [44], neurotransmitter activities [45, 46], and various other integrating hormonal systems [47–49].

Various types of stress such as cold and hot exposures, social crowding and handling, as well as age and a diabetic condition may lead to a reduced number of receptors for adrenal steroids in hippocampus. A common factor in these conditions is the persistent elevation of corticosterone in the circulation [11]. There is a downregulation of glucocorticoid receptors with the elevated level of corticosterone [6]. The regulation of corticosterone receptors shows a biphasic increase with adrenalectomy. In the first 12–18 h after bilateral adrenalectomy, the rise is mainly due to clearance of endogenous hormone. The second phase takes a number of days to develop fully and represents an increase in total receptor numbers [50]. The initial increase in binding sites is relatively constant for 3–4 days postadrenalectomy. Binding then rises up to 30 days when it returns to 3-day level and finally falls still further when measured 180 days after the operation [51]. The number of hippocampal glucocorticoid binding sites is reduced by injecting corticosterone into adrenalectomized rats [52].

Brain glucocorticoid receptors also respond to chronic stress-induced elevations of circulating corticosteroids [53]. Repeated stress over 3 weeks decreases the number of cytosolic receptors in the hippocampus. This up- and downregulation of glucocorticoid receptors in some brain regions and pituitary is thought to be governed not only by corticosteroids but also by certain neuropeptides such as vasopressin and ACTH [46, 49].

By the 14th postoperative day, hypophysectomy increases the retention of labeled corticosterone by nuclei of in vivo cells more than adrenalectomy. Cytosolic [^{3}H]corticosterone binding at 14 days is also higher in the hippocampus, hypothalamus, and septum of hypophysectomized rats. This binding is reversible by systemic administration of corticosterone and ACTH [46].

A main action of glucocorticoids on the brain and pituitary is to govern the production and secretion of hormones of the hypothalamic-pituitary-adrenal axis [11]. The feedback actions of adrenal steroids have been categorized into three groups: fast, intermediate, and slow [13]. The first category involves the direct actions of glucocorticoids on the membranes, independent of RNA and protein synthesis, to change blood steroid levels. The second category involves actions of glucocorticoids which influence

RNA and protein synthesis and which regulate gene expression related to cellular and metabolic events. The third category involves actions of glucocorticoids that suppress the synthesis of CRH, vasopressin and ACTH; these actions also involve RNA and protein synthesis and are responsible for the negative feedback of glucocorticoids on hypothalamus and pituitary [13].

The negative feedback actions of glucocorticoids affect not only the hypothalamus and pituitary but also the hippocampus, amygdala, septum and midbrain. For example, ablation of dorsal hippocampus reduces the effectiveness of dexamethasone in inhibiting basal and stress-induced pituitary-adrenal responses [54]. Because the stress response is lowered when hippocampal neurons are irreversibly lost and also by reduction in number of hippocampal corticosterone receptors [55], the hippocampus is thought to be a site for negative feedback by corticosterone in shutdown of the stress response. This reduction in receptor numbers is very specific for the hippocampus and does not occur in pituitary, hypothalamus, amygdala or septum, and restoration of normal receptor levels leads to reversal of the stress shutoff. However, in case of aging rats, the receptor deficit is due to neuronal loss [48].

The exact mechanism of hippocampal neurotoxicity by glucocorticoids is not well understood. It appears that age-related loss of hippocampal neurons is caused by cumulative exposure to basal titers of the steroid and that prolonged stress can accelerate such hippocampal aging [56]. Glucocorticoids have long been recognized for their potent catabolic effects on target tissues which include inhibition of glucose uptake, cell division, protein synthesis, as well as depletion of glycogen and triglycerides [7]. Thus, cumulative exposure to glucocorticoids as a function of age may ultimately prove sufficiently catabolic to directly destroy hippocampal neurons. On the other hand, glucocorticoid-induced neuronal loss may also occur in conjunction with other metabolic challenges with aging.

There are several pathological repercussions of the corticosterone hypersecretion in the aged rats. Most severe is the progressive loss of hippocampal neurons with prolonged exposure to corticosterone. This neuronal loss appears to accelerate further corticosterone secretion and shows a feed forward cascade with age. This would enhance the neuronal degeneration in the hippocampus and lead to hyperadrenocorticism [6]. Another consequence may be the reduced sprouting of axons. This phenomenon is produced in younger rats by maintaining corticosterone at high levels [57]. Elevated cortisone levels apparently have more widespread consequences outside of the brain. For example, stress induces tumor growth in both young and old rats [58] but with increased incidence in the aged rats. This may in part be due to higher glucocorticoid levels in aged rats [58]. Also, glucocorticoid increase may be a causative factor in immunosuppression, hypertension, osteoporosis and steroid diabetes with advancing age [7].

Conclusions

The brain possesses receptors for adrenal glucocorticoids which change in number and some physicochemical properties during development and aging. Glucocorticoids affect several neurochemical reactions within the brain, including monoamines, amino acid transmitters, and some neuropeptides such as CRH, vasopressin, and ACTH. Their biochemical effects include regulation of neurotransmitter receptor levels, production of second messengers, and induction of several enzymes. Efficient functioning of the hypothalamic-pituitary-adrenal axis appears to be essential for adrenocortical stress reponses on and off. In general, the efficiency of this axis becomes reduced as a function of age, which may lead to decreased adaptive response in aged animals. Repeated exposure to various kinds of stresses throughout the life span induces alterations which depend on age and target tissue. These alterations may disrupt appropriate articulation and timing of the necessary signals for an optimal hypothalamic-pituitary-adrenocortical function and thereby prevent efficient adjustments to internal and external demands as a function of age.

References

1 Timiras, P.S.: Physiology of ageing: aspects of neuroendocrine regulation; in Pathy, Principles and practice of geriatric medicine (Wiley, Chichester 1985).

2 Finch, C.E.; Landfield, P.W.: Neuroendocrine and autonomic functions in aging mammals; in Finch, Schneider, Handbook of the biology of aging; 2nd ed. (Van Nostrand & Reinhold, New York 1985).

3 Meites, J.: Changes in hypothalamic regulation of pituitary function in aging rats; in Enna, Samorajski, Beer, Brain neurotransmitters and receptors and aging and age-related disorders (Raven Press, New York 1981).

4 Cannon, W.G.: Organization of physiological homeostasis. Physiol. Rev. *9:* 399–431 (1929).

5 Selye, M.; Prioreschi, P.: Stress theory of aging; in Shock, Aging – some social and biological aspects (American Association of Advanced Science, Washington 1960).

6 Sapolsky, R.M.; Krey, L.C.; McEwen, B.S.: The neuroendocrinology of stress and aging: the glucocorticoid cascade hypothesis. Endocr. Rev. *7:* 284–301 (1986).
7 Munck, A.; Guyre, P.M.; Holbrook, N.J.: Physiological functions of glucocorticoids in stress and their relation to pharmacological actions. Endocr. Rev. *5:* 25–44 (1984).
8 Makara, G.B.: Mechanisms by which stressful stimuli activate the pituitary-adrenal system. Fed. Proc. *44:* 149–153 (1985).
9 McEwen, B.S.: Glucocorticoids and hippocampus: receptors in search of a function; in Ganten, Pfaff, Current topics in neuroendocrinology, pp. 1–22 (Springer, Berlin 1982).
10 Meyer, J.S.: Biochemical effects of corticosteroids in neural tissues. Physiol. Rev. *65:* 946–1020 (1985).
11 McEwen, B.S.; Kloet, E.R.; Rostene, W.: Adrenal steroid receptors and actions in the nervous system. Physiol. Rev. *66:* 1121–1188 (1986).
12 Nakajima, S.: Hippocampal protein synthesis and spike discharges in relation to memory; in Isaacson, Pribram, The hippocampus vol. 1, pp. 393–413 (Plenum Press, New York 1975).
13 Keller-Wood, M.E.; Dallman, M.F.: Corticosteroid inhibition of ACTH secretion. Endocr. Rev. *5:* 1–24 (1984).
14 Alexis, M.N.; Stylianopoulou, F.; Kitraki, E.; Sekeris, C.E.: The distribution and properties of the glucocorticoid receptor from the rat brain and pituitary. J. biol. Chem. *258:* 4710–4714 (1983).
15 Meyer, J.S.; McEwen, B.S.: Evidence for glucocorticoid target cells in the rat optic nerve. Physicochemical characterization of cytosol binding sites. J. Neurochem. *39:* 435–442 (1982).
16 Clark, C.R.; MacLusky, N.J.; Naftolin, F.: Glucocorticoid receptors in the spinal cord. Brain Res. *217:* 412–415 (1981).
17 Yamamoto, K.R.A.: Steroid receptor regulated transcription of specific genes and gene networks. A. Rev. Genet. *19:* 209–252 (1985).
18 Kalimi, M.; Beato, M.; Feigelson, P.: Interaction of glucocorticoids with rat liver nuclei. I. Role of cytosol proteins. Biochemistry *12:* 3365–3371 (1973).
19 Milgrom, E.; Atger, M.; Baulieu, E.E.: Audiophilic activation of steroid hormone receptors, Biochemistry *12:* 5198–5205 (1973).
20 Bailly, A.; Savouret, J.F.; Sallas, N.; Milgrom, E.: Factors modifying the equilibrium between activated and non-activated forms of steroid-receptor complexes. Eur. J. Biochem. *88:* 623–632 (1978).
21 Disorbo, D.M.; Phelps, D.S.; Litwack, G.: Chemical probes of amino acid residues affect the active sites of the glucocorticoid receptors. Endocrinology *106:* 922–929 (1980).
22 Munck, A.; Foley, R.: Activation of steroid hormone-receptor complexes in intact target cells in physiological conditions. Nature *278:* 752–754 (1979).
23 Markovic, R.D.; Litwack, G.: Activation of liver and kidney glucocorticoid-receptor complexes occurs in vivo. Archs Biochem. Biophys. *202:* 374–379 (1980).
24 Kanungo, M.S.: Changes in enzymes during ageing; in Biochemistry of ageing, pp. 79–126 (Academic Press, London 1980).
25 Roth, G.S.; Hess, G.: Changes in the mechanisms of hormone and neurotransmitter

action during aging: current status of the role of receptor and post-receptor alterations. Mech. Age. Dev. *20:* 175–194 (1982).

26 Kalimi, M.: Glucocorticoid receptors: from development to aging. A review. Mech. Age. Dev. *24:* 129–138 (1984).

27 Olpe, H.R.; McEwen, B.S.: Glucocorticoid binding to receptor-like proteins in rat brains and pituitary: ontogenetic and experimentally induced changes. Brain Res. *105:* 121–128 (1976).

28 Clayton, C.J.; Grosser, R.I.; Stevens, W.: The ontogeny of corticosterone and dexamethasone receptors in rat brain. Brain Res. *134:* 445–453 (1977).

29 Kitraki, E.; Alexis, M.N.; Stylianopoulou, F.: Glucocorticoid receptors in developing rat brain and liver. J. Steroid Biochem. *20:* 263–269 (1984).

30 Sharma, R.; Timiras, P.S.: Regulatory changes in glucocorticoid receptors in the skeletal muscle of immature and mature male rats. Mech. Age. Dev. *37:* 248–256 (1987).

31 Sharma, R.; Timiras, P.S.: Age-dependent regulation of glucocorticoid receptors in the liver of male rats. Biochim. biophys. Acta (in press).

32 Salky, M.; Koch, B.: Physicochemical analysis of glucocorticoid receptors in the immature pituitary gland: evidence for lability and aggregation of the heat-activated form. Mol. cell. Endocrinol. *28:* 27–35 (1982).

33 Salky, M.; Koch, B.: Ontogenesis of glucocorticoid receptors in anterior pituitary gland: transient dissociation among cytosolic receptor density, nuclear uptake and regulation of corticotropic activity. Endocrinology *108:* 591–596 (1981).

34 Sharma, R.; Timiras, P.S.: Activation of glucocorticoid receptors in the cerebral hemispheres of weanling and adult male rats. INS-ASN Joint Meet. Neurochem., La Guaira 1987).

35 Sapolsky, R.M.; Meaney, M.J.: Maturation of the adrenocortical stress response: neuroendocrine control mechanisms and the stress hyporesponsive period. Brain Res. Rev. *11:* 65–76 (1986).

36 Roth, G.S.: Age-related changes in specific glucocorticoid binding by steroid-responsive tissues of rats. Endocrinology *94:* 82–90 (1974).

37 Roth, G.S.: Reduced glucocorticoid binding site concentration in cortical neuronal perikarya from senescent rats. Brain Res. *107:* 345–354 (1976).

38 Sharma, R.; Timiras, P.S.: Changes in glucocorticoid receptors in different regions of brain of immature and mature male rats. Biochem. int. *13:* 609–614 (1986).

39 Neuben, J.; Holinka, C.; Latham, K.; Allen, J.; Finch, C.: Corticosterone binding in cytosols from brain regions of mature and senescent male C57BL/6J mice. Brain. Res. *115:* 345-351 (1976).

40 Defoire, C.; Turner, B.: Glucocorticoid binding is decreased in hippocampus but not cortex of aged rats. Abstr. Soc. Neurosci. *7:* 947 (1981).

41 Sapolsky, R.M.; Krey, L.C.; McEwen, B.S.: Corticosterone receptors decline in a site-specific manner in the aged rat brain. Brain Res. *289:* 235–240 (1983).

42 Meaney, M.J.; Sapolsky, R.M.; McEwen, B.S.: The development of the glucocorticoid receptor system in the rat limbic brain. II. An autoradiographic study. Devl. Brain Res. *18:* 165–168 (1985).

43 Muhlen, K.A.A.D.; Ockenfels, H.: Morphologische Veränderungen im Diencephalon und Telencephalon: Störungen des Regelkreises Adenohypophysennebennierenrinde. Z. Zellforsch. mikrosk. Anat. *93:* 126–141 (1969).

44 Nyakas, C.; Dekloet, E.R.; Veldhuis, M.D.; Bohus, B.: Corticosterone binding capacity increases in contralateral hippocampus after partial unilateral hippocampectomy. Neurosci. Lett. *21:* 339–343 (1981).
45 Valery, P.; Palmery, M.; Patacchioli, F.R.; Catalani, A.; Tita, B.; Angelucci, L.: Role and regulation of brain glucocorticoid receptors. Pharmacol. Res. Commun. *12:* 283–292 (1980).
46 Veldhuis, M.D.; Dekloet, E.R.: Significance of ACTH (4–10) in the control of hippocampal corticosterone receptor capacity of hypophysectomized rats. Neuroendocrinology *34:* 374–380 (1982).
47 Fridman, O.; Foglia, V.G.; DeNicola, A.F.: Reduction of [^{3}H]corticosterone binding to cytoplasmic receptors in the brain of diabetic rats. J. Steroid Biochem. *9:* 609–614 (1978).
48 Sapolsky, R.M.; Krey, L.C.; McEwen, B.S.; Rainbow, T.C.: Do vasopressin-related peptides induce hippocampal corticosterone receptors? Implications for Aging. J. Neurosci. *4:* 1479–1485 (1984).
49 Veldhuis, M.D.; Dekloet, E.R.: Vasopressin-related peptides increase the hippocampal corticosterone receptor capacity of diabetes insipidus (Brattleboro rat). Endocrinology *110:* 153–157 (1982).
50 McEwen, B.S.; Wallach, G.; Magnus, C.: Corticosterone binding to hippocampus: immediate and delayed influences of the absence of adrenal secretion. Brain Res. *70:* 321–334 (1974).
51 Stevens, W.; Reed, D.J.; Grosser, B.I.: Binding of natural and synthetic glucocorticoids in rat brain. J. Steroid Biochem. *6:* 521–527 (1975).
52 Tornello, S.; Orti, E.; DeNicola, A.F.; Rainbow, T.C.; McEwen, B.S.: Regulation of glucocorticoid receptors in brain by corticosterone treatment of adrenalectomized rats. Neuroendocrinology *35:* 411–417 (1982).
53 Sapolsky, R.M.; Krey, L.C.; McEwen, B.S.: Stress down-regulates corticosterone receptors in a site specific manner in the brain. Endocrinology *114:* 287–292 (1984).
54 Feldman, S.; Conforti, N.: Participation of the dorsal hippocampus in the glucocorticoid feedback effect on adrenocortical activity. Neuroendocrinology *30:* 52–55 (1980).
55 Sapolsky, R.M.; Krey, L.C.; McEwen, B.S.: Glucocorticoid-sensitive hippocampal neurons are involved in terminating the adrenocortical stress response. Proc. natn. Acad. Sci. USA *81:* 6174–6177 (1984).
56 Sapolsky, R.M.; Krey, L.C.; McEwen, B.S.: The adrenocortical stress response in the aged male rat: impairment of recovery from stress. Exp. Gerontol. *18:* 55–63 (1983).
57 Dekosky, S.T.; Scheff, S.W.; Cotman, C.W.: Elevated corticosterone levels. A possible cause of reduced axon sprouting in aged animals. Neuroendocrinology *38:* 33–38 (1984).
58 Sapolsky, R.M.; Donnelly, T.M.: Vulnerability to stress-induced tumor growth increases with age in rats: role of glucocorticoids. Endocrinology *117:* 662–666 (1985).

Dr. Paola S. Timiras, Department of Physiology-Anatomy,
University of California, Berkeley, CA 94720 (USA)

Interdiscipl. Topics Geront., vol. 24, pp. 111–124 (Karger, Basel 1988)

Decline in Growth Hormone Secretion in Aging Animals and Man

William E. Sonntag[a], *Joseph Meites*[b, 1]

[a] Department of Physiology and Pharmacology, Bowman Gray School of Medicine of Wake Forest University, Winston-Salem, N.C., USA;
[b] Department of Physiology, Neuroendocrine Research Laboratory, Michigan State University, East Lansing, Mich., USA

Introduction

It is well known that aging in mammals is characterized by a general reduction in function of many tissues and organs, a decline in immune function, and diminished lean body mass. Current theories of aging suggest that at least some of the changes in tissue function may be the result of a decline in anabolic hormones which normally serve to stimulate these tissues. Growth hormone (GH) is the most important protein anabolic agent in the body and appears to be essential for protein synthesis throughout life. This hormone also promotes bone growth, functions of the liver, kidney, and hematopoietic system, and has been implicated as an important regulator of immunological vigor. GH also importantly influences carbohydrate, lipid, vitamin, and mineral metabolism. The close similarity between several characteristic changes that occur with age and the biological actions of GH have led us to hypothesize that the decline in the function of many tissues with age is the result, at least in part, of diminished GH secretion [52].

The purpose of this chapter is to review (a) evidence for a decline in GH secretion with age, (b) the neuroendrocrine mechanisms responsible

[1] The authors wish to express their appreciation to Dr. Victoria Kingsbury for her editorial assistance in the preparation of the manuscript. This work was supported in part by NIH grants AG05637 and AG04207 (to WES) and AG00416 (to JM).

for the decrease in GH secretion, and (c) evidence that GH is at least partly responsible for the decline in thymic function and protein synthesis – two systems which classically have been reported to deteriorate with age.

GH, Somatomedin-C

Much of the earlier work on plasma or serum GH levels with age was controversial because only single samples of blood were assayed. However, it was noted in young men that GH was secreted in discrete pulses, primarily after the onset of sleep [42, 54]. Several other studies reported that the amplitude of GH pulses appeared to decline with increasing age [6, 10, 37, 41]. In 1976, Tannenbaum and Martin [56] reported that in rats GH was secreted in large pulses at 3- to 4-hour intervals throughout the day. In their study, GH levels were observed to range from less than 10 ng/ml to greater than 600 ng/ml over a time period as brief as 20 min. Subsequently, our laboratory reported that the amplitude of GH pulses was greatly reduced in old as compared to young male rats [52]. In this study, GH pulse amplitude in the old rats declined by approximately 50% as did pituitary GH content. The amplitude of the majority of GH pulses in the old animals averaged less than 200 ng/ml whereas in young animals the average amplitude was consistently greater than 400 ng/ml. There appeared to be no changes in basal or trough concentrations of GH. Furthermore, these changes did not appear to be related to increased GH inactivation since studies revealed that GH metabolism is unchanged in old male [Sonntag, unpubl. observations] and female rats [16].

The significance of the lower amplitude of the GH pulses in male rats, in our opinion, was that (a) these changes appeared to be identical to those reported in man, suggesting that this decline may be a basic mechanism of mammalian aging, with functional significance, and (b) the mechanism for the decline in GH pulses could be investigated more thoroughly by using an animal model.

The decline in the amplitude of pulsatile GH release with age has been widely confirmed in a number of different animal models used in aging research. Kahler et al. [22], for example, reported a decline in the amplitude and mean concentrations of GH in rhesus monkeys over a 24-hour period. More recently, Takahashi et al. [53] reported a decline in the amplitude of growth hormone release in aging female rats (fig. 1). A significant finding in this study was that the decline in GH secretion occurred as

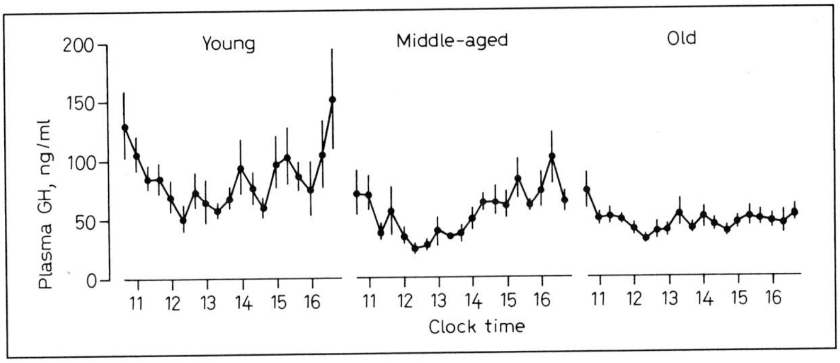

Fig. 1. Mean plasma GH concentrations in young, middle-aged, and old female rats. Each point represents mean GH levels in 17 young, 6 middle-aged, and 13 old rats [with permission, 53].

early as 11 months of age with a concomitant decline in pituitary GH content [14]. The authors suggested that the early decrease in GH secretion may account for the early body growth stasis observed in female rats. Similar results were recently reported in postmenopausal women 57–76 years of age. There was a decline in the proportion of large pulses and a corresponding increase in the numbers of small pulses compared to younger women [19]. These results strongly suggest that the decline in amplitude of GH pulses is characteristic of aging mammals and may have a causal relationship to the decline in many tissue functions with age.

For several years, it was recognized that the majority of the effects of GH are mediated through the actions of somatomedin-C (also termed insulin-like growth factor-1) [8]. Although somatomedin-C is found in many tissues and organs as well as in fibroblasts, this hormone is most abundant in the perisinusoidal capillaries of the liver, and it seems likely that plasma levels of the hormone are primarily regulated by secretion from this tissue [18]. It has been clearly established that, with increasing age, there is a progressive reduction in plasma levels of somatomedin-C in rats when measured either by radioreceptor or radioimmunoassay [11, 13]. Studies of age-related changes in somatomedin-C levels in man by a number of investigators have also revealed a significant decline with age [19, 21, 41]. Florini et al. [12] suggested that the decline in somatomedin-C results from the reduction in integrated concentrations of GH in the plasma. However, in another study, direct statistical comparisons between the two variables revealed that the fraction of GH secreted in pulses had the strongest correlation with plasma levels of somatomedin-C [19]. Nevertheless, it is clear that the declines in plasma levels of somatomedin-C are secondary to age-related changes in some aspect of GH secretion since GH administration to older individuals increases plasma levels of somatomedin-C [21].

Growth-Hormone-Releasing Factor

All possible causes for the reduction in pulsatile release of GH have not been completely determined. Previous studies have indicated that GH content in the pituitary gland declines by 18 months of age in male rats [52] and by 11 months of age in female rats [53]. Although it was reported that there were no differences in the ability of growth-hormone-releasing factor (GRF) to stimulate GH release in vivo in 3- to 4- and 19- to 21-month-old male rats [61], studies in our own as well as other laboratories have suggested that the capacity of GRF to stimulate GH release in vivo declines with advancing age [7, 50]. The decline in GRF-induced release of GH has also been confirmed in elderly men [44], and the data suggest that some aspect of GRF-mediated GH release is altered with age and may be responsible for the decline in pulsatile release of GH.

Although the in vivo data on the GH response to GRF with age appear to be relatively consistent, there seems to be some controversy as to whether the mechanism for this decline is primarily related to diminished pituitary response to GRF or is secondary to other age-associated phenomena (e.g. increased somatostatin release). By using a pituitary slice preparation in vitro, Sonntag et al. [50] demonstrated similar capacities of pituitary tissue from young and old rats to secrete GH in response to GRF. Young and old male Sprague-Dawley rats demonstrated a 30 and 74% increase in GH release in response to 10^{-9} and 10^{-7} *M* GRF, respectively. Our results clearly suggest that the reduced response to GRF in vivo does not result from a diminished response to GRF but from the influence of other hypothalamic factors being released, probably increased somatostatin from hypothalamic neurons. This conclusion is consistent with an earlier study published by our laboratory demonstrating that passive immunization with somatostatin antiserum increased GH release as much or more in old than in young rats [46]. However, our in vitro results have been challenged by another study in which the pituitary response to GRF in young and old rats was assessed by using cultured dispersed pituitary cells [7]. In response to 2 h of stimulation with synthetic rat GRF, the authors reported a diminished increase in GH release in old as compared to young rats, and an attenuated rise in cAMP production by the pituitaries of the older rats. Besides the differences in tissue preparation, at least another major difference between these studies was the length of time the tissue was stimulated with GRF. Previous studies have demonstrated that GRF stimulates GH synthesis as well as release, and it is possible that these two cellular processes may be differentially affected by aging. We have reconfirmed our original in vivo results on the age-related decline of GH release in response to GRF, and assessed the effects of GRF in vitro on pituitary slices in a superfusion system using stimulation periods as brief as 1 min [49]. Our results clearly demonstrate that there is no loss in sensitivity to GRF with age. GRF administration produced parallel dose response curves in pituitary tissues from young, middle-aged, and old rats when data were expressed as percent increase from baseline. We concluded that the deficiency in GH release in old animals does not result from a deficiency in the capacity of GRF to stimulate GH release, but rather is due to decreased ability of the somatotrophs to synthesize GH.

Somatostatin

Although the mechanisms for the alteration in pituitary response to GRF with age remain to be established, recent data have implicated alterations in the release of somatostatin from hypothalamic neurons as an important factor in the decline in GH pulses during aging in the rat. Previous research has indicated that the only stimulus capable of increasing GH release to the same degree in young and old rats is passive immunization with somatostatin antiserum [46]. Depending on the dose of antiserum, the increase in GH release was actually greater in old than in young rats. These results suggest that GH release in old rats is either tonically inhibited by somatostatin or that the somatotrophs of aging rats are more sensitive to the inhibitory effects of somatostatin.

We have studied hypothalamic somatostatin release directly from median eminence fragments of young and old male Sprague-Dawley rats by stimulating these tissues with 55 mM K^+ in vitro [48]. In all cases, tissues from aging rats exhibited a greater fractional efflux of somatostatin than tissues from young rats. Somatostatin is known to exist in two biologically active forms, somatostatin-14 and somatostatin-28. Although somatostatin-28 appears to be a precursor for the -14 form of the peptide, somatostatin-28 may have a distinct role in the regulation of pituitary GH release since the biological activity of this peptide is greater than somatostatin-14 on a molar basis [55]. When we compared the fractional efflux of each of these peptides, the release of somatostatin-14 was unchanged with age whereas the release of the -28 form of the peptide was greater in old rats. These results suggest that the increases in biological activity of somatostatin, possibly as a result of alterations in posttranslational processing of the molecule, are partly responsible for the decline in GH pulses, plasma levels of somatomedin-C, and subsequently in protein synthetic capacity of old rats.

Neural Regulation of GH Secretion

GH secretion is regulated by both neurotransmitters and neuropeptides which control the release of somatostatin and GRF from hypothalamic neurons [32]. For example, norepinephrine (NE) and dopamine (DA) or synthetic agonists of these compounds have all been shown to stimulate the release of GH in animals [23, 35, 58] and man [3, 26, 33], whereas antagonists inhibit GH release. Similarly, endogenous opioid peptides, which are found in high concentrations in the brain, produce a rapid elevation of GH release which can be antagonized by the opiate receptor blocker, naloxone [4, 9, 30, 43]. However, there is some controversy about whether opioid peptides participate in the physiological regulation of GH release since naloxone appears to have no effect on the basal secretion of GH in the rat [57]. In man, enkephalin analogs have been reported to increase GH secretion [17]. However, in contrast to the rat, naloxone administration decreased GH release induced by arginine infusion or exercise stress, but failed to reduce basal levels of GH or to abolish the rise in GH produced by apomorphine, *L*-dopa, insulin hypoglycemia, or sleep [27, 31, 34, 60]. These observations further indicate that there are important differences in the neural regulation of GH secretion between animals and man.

We have tested the capacity of several CNS-active drugs to increase GH release in young and old animals [46]. The α-adrenergic receptor agonist, clonidine, the dopamine receptor agonist, piribedil, and morphine produced a smaller increase in GH release in old than in young male rats. Similar results were found in old female rats after administration of clonidine or morphine. In elderly men, there are also reports of diminished GH release after *L*-dopa administration, exercise [1], or insulin-induced hypoglycemia [28]. Although the specific causes for these differences are unknown, the diminished capacity to increase GH release in response to pharmacological stimuli with age may be the result of (a) diminished neurotransmitter receptors, (b) inadequate release of GRF, (c) failure to inhibit somatostatin secretion, or (d) altered pituitary response to GRF and/or somatostatin.

Many of the neuroendocrine changes that occur in aging animals are the result of alterations in the synthesis and release of neurotransmitters. It is well established that the content and turnover of the hypothalamic catecholamines (CAs), DA, and NE are reduced in old rats, whereas the turnover of serotonin is unchanged or slightly increased [20, 45]. Similar changes in hypothalamic CAs have been reported to occur in elderly humans. It is possible to assess whether hypothalamic CAs are involved in the aging process by treatment of old rats with the CA precursor, *L*-dopa, which has been shown to increase the turnover of DA and NE. Using this paradigm, we have demonstrated that treatment of old male rats with *L*-dopa for 8 days restored high amplitude GH pulses and mean GH concentrations to levels comparable to those in young animals [47]. Treatment of old animals with vehicle revealed the characteristic reduction in amplitude of GH pulses with age. These results clearly demonstrate that hypothalamic CAs are important factors in the reduction in amplitude of GH pulses and, by their action on somatostatin and/or GRF neurons, are responsible for the decline in GH secretion with age.

Feedback on Hypothalamic Neurons

It has been well established that one of the mechanisms that regulates GH release from the anterior pituitary includes feedback from plasma levels of somatomedin-C and GH [2, 39]. It has been established that this feedback occurs directly on the somatotrophs (in the case of somatomedin-C), and by regulating release of somatostatin and possibly GRF from hypothalamic neurons. Although little information on the effects of GH and somatomedin-C on GRF release is available, these hormones clearly have the potential to promote somatostatin release into the hypophysial portal blood, thereby lowering plasma levels of GH. Since both plasma levels of GH and somatomedin-C decline with age, it is likely that the decline in the amplitude of GH pulses is related to (a) inability of hypothalamic neurons to detect the decrease in plasma levels of these hormones, (b) diminished ability to stimulate GRF release and/or inhibition of somatostatin release in response to appropriate stimuli, or (c) alterations in the synthesis and/or release of GH at the level of the pituitary gland. The results reported to date suggest an integral role for hypothalamic CAs in this feedback process, but the specific mechanisms involved are unknown.

Steroid and Thyroid Hormones

Early studies suggested that several steroid and thyroid hormones influenced pituitary secretion of GH. Thyroid hormones, estrogens, and corticosteroids were all implicated as important regulators of GH release. However, there have been few studies on the influence of steroid hormones on pulsatile GH release and only one study, to our knowledge, on the interaction of estrogen with pulsatile GH release. In a very detailed analysis of pulsatile GH release in men and women, Ho et al. [19] reported that the decline in large-amplitude GH pulses with age was correlated most closely with decreases in free estradiol levels. The authors concluded that free estradiol amplifies GH pulses and that at least part of the age-related decline in GH secretion resulted from decreases in estradiol secretion. No effects of testosterone on the amplitude of GH secretion were observed, although the authors detected an independent influence of age on circulating GH concentrations. Thyroid hormones were reported to influence GH secretion, but the possible influences of thyroid hormones (or adrenal steroids) on GH secretion with age remain to be determined.

Implications of Diminished GH Secretion with Age

Thymic Function

It is well known that thymic size and T cell function decline with age. Many investigators have reported diminished T cell proliferative responses to mitogens, reduced serum levels of thymic hormones, and lower secretion of interleukin-2 in old animals as compared to these values in young animals [29, 59]. The decline in T cell proliferation is preceded by thymic atrophy, and thymic implants or thymic hormone administration were reported to partially restore the diminished T cell proliferation that normally occurs during aging [15, 63]. These results have led several investigators to suggest that the thymus gland is a key component of immunological aging, although the specific mechanisms responsible for these age-related alterations are unknown. Several hypotheses for the decline in T cell function have been suggested, including (a) clonal exhaustion of progenitor T cells in the bone marrow that migrate into the thymus, (b) alterations in DNA within the thymocytes, and (c) a decline in extrinsic or trophic-hormonal factors [24]. This later hypothesis appears most tenable since it is well known that thymic size and GH secretion from the anterior pituitary gland are maximal at puberty and decline thereafter [62]. Furthermore, treatment of young animals with pituitary extracts or GH was reported to enhance thymic size [40]. Recent evidence has also suggested that treatment of 16- and 22-month-old female Wistar-Furth rats for 2 months with GH_3 pituitary adenoma cells, which secrete both GH and prolactin, increased thymic size, and T cell proliferative responses of splenocytes from implanted rats 2- to 5-fold more than in 18-month-old controls [25]. Furthermore, splenocytes from 24-month-old GH_3-implanted rats showed augmented T cell proliferative responses and increased synthesis of interleukin-2 when compared to values in controls. Although this report did not distinguish between the effects of GH and prolactin, the data provide strong evidence that alterations in neuroendocrine function can modify immunological aging.

Protein Synthesis

The age-related decline in protein synthesis in skeletal muscle and liver appears to be another biochemical correlate of the aging process. In many tissues, there is a progressive reduction in total protein synthetic activity with age, including declines in kidney, liver, brain, skeletal, and cardiac muscle [38]. Several investigators have suggested that this decline is related to a reduction in poly-A+ RNA synthesis, which would indicate that deficiencies in transcription of DNA are at least partly responsible for these age-related deficits. More recently, however, Pluskal et al. [36] have reported a 40% decline in the activity of polyribosomes prepared from old as compared to young animals using a cell-free system. In addition, there appeared to be a decline in the activity of soluble factors in the pH 5 enzyme fraction prepared from 12- and 22- to 24-month-old rats. These results suggested that not only is there a progressive age-related decline in levels of mRNA in the tissues of aged rats but that the efficiency of the ribosome protein factor complex necessary to initiate and maintain protein synthesis is reduced with age. Further studies suggested that the decline in polysome activity in aged animals may be due to changes in the activity of initiation/elongation factors in the nonribosomal protein fractions of the cell [5]. Since these factors are essential for translation of mRNA into protein, it was hypothesized that reduction in these proteins, together with the decline in mRNA levels, contributes to the general reduction in protein synthesis in skeletal muscle with age.

In an effort to test whether extrinsic or hormonal factors are responsible for the deficits in protein synthetic capacity with age, we recently assessed the ability of exogenous GH to increase protein synthesis in aging animals. We found that administration of bovine GH to male Sprague-Dawley rats increased the rate of ^{3}H-phenylalanine incorporation into total protein and the rate of protein synthesis after correction for the intracellular leucine-specific activity [51]. We hypothesized that GH stimulates transcription of DNA and/or translational processes in aging rats since the changes in relative rates of protein synthesis did not appear to result from increased ^{3}H-phenylalanine uptake or alteration in the intracellular phenylalanine-specific activity. Our results are consistent with previous data in which GH administration was shown to increase heart, liver, kidney, and spleen weight in old rats, thymus weight in aged mice [32], and somatomedin-C levels in elderly humans [12]. Although increases in organ weight or protein synthesis are not necessarily indicative of improved tissue function, these results clearly demonstrate that some aspect of the age-related decline in protein synthesis may not be the result of intrinsic changes within tissues but result from changes in hormone secretion.

Conclusions – GH as a Model for Aging of the Neuroendocrine System

The studies on GH to date clearly indicate that a decline in the amplitude of GH pulses is a characteristic feature of mammalian aging. Many studies in rodents and primates, including man, support this conclusion. Age-related declines in GH secretion are one of the few neuroendocrine variables that consistently change with age in a number of different species. This cross-species consistency provides a basis for use of GH changes in secretion as a model for studies on aging of the neuroendocrine system. Investigation of the mechanisms responsible for these changes in GH secretion in rats is likely to point to similar control in other species. Furthermore, the age-related changes in GH secretion appear to have direct consequences on plasma levels of somatomedin-C, protein synthesis, and immune function. Although little information is currently available on the relation between the decline in GH secretion and bone loss during aging, it is possible that the reduced GH secretion is also partly responsible for increased bone loss. Whether treatment with GH or agents that increase GH secretion can improve various body functions during aging remains to be investigated.

References

1 Bazarre, T.; Johanson, S.; Huseman, C.; Varma, M.; Blizzard, R.: Human growth hormone changes with age. Proc. 3rd Int. Symp. Growth Hormone, Milan North Amsterdam 1978.

2 Berelowitz, M.; Szabo, M.; Frohman, L.; Fierstone, S.; Chu, L.: Somatomedin-C mediates growth hormone negative feedback by effects on both the hypothalamus and pituitary. Science *212:* 1279–1281 (1981).

3 Boyd, A.; Lebovitz, H.; Pfeiffer, J.: Stimulation of human growth hormone secretion with *L*-Dopa. New Engl. J. Med. *283:* 1425–1428 (1970).

4 Bruni, J.; Van Vugt, D.; Marshall, S.; Meites, J.: Effects of naloxone, morphine, and methionine enkephalin on serum prolactin, luteinizing hormone, follicle stimulating hormone, thyroid stimulating hormone and growth hormone. Life Sci. *21:* 461–466 (1977).

5 Burini, R.; Pluskal, M.; Wei, I.; Young, V.: Protein synthesis studies in skeletal muscle of aging rats. II. In vitro studies with 0.5 *M* potassium chloride washed polyribosomes. J. Geront. *39:* 392–397 (1984).

6 Carlson, H.; Gillin, J.; Gorden, P.; Snyder, F.: Absence of sleep-related growth hormone peaks in aged normal subjects and in acromegaly. J. clin. Endocr. Metab. *34:* 1102–1107 (1972).

7 Ceda, G.; Valenti, G.; Butterini, U.; Hoffman, A.: Diminished pituitary response to growth hormone releasing factor in aging male rats. Endocrinology *118:* 2109–2114 (1986).

8 Daughaday, W.; Hall, K.; Raben, M.; Salmon, W.; Vanden Brande, L.; Van Wyk, J.: Somatomedin: proposed designation for sulfation factor. Nature *235:* 107–109 (1972).

9 Dupont, A.; Cusan, L.; Garon, M.; Labrie, F.; Li, C.: B-Endorphin: stimulation of growth hormone release in vitro. Proc. natn. Acad. Sci. *74:* 358–359 (1977).

10 Finkelstein, J.; Roffwarg, H.; Boyar, R.; Kream, J.; Hellman, L.: Age-related changes in the twenty-four hour spontaneous secretion of growth hormone. J. clin. Endocr. Metab. *35:* 665–670 (1972).

11 Florini, J.; Harned, J.; Richman, R.; Weiss, J.: Effect of rat age on serum levels of growth hormone and somatomedins. Mech. Age. Dev. *15:* 165–176 (1981).

12 Florini, J.; Prinz, P.; Vitiello, M.; Hintz, R.: Somatomedin-C levels in healthy young and old men: relationship to peak and 24-hour integrated levels of GH. J. Geront. *40:* 2–7 (1985).

13 Florini, J.; Roberts, S.: Effects of rat age on blood levels of somatomedin-like growth factor. J. Geront. *35:* 23–30 (1979).

14 Forman, L.; Sonntag, W.; Hylka, V.; Meites, J.: Pituitary growth hormone and hypothalamic somatostatin in young female rats versus old constant estrous female rats. Experientia *41:* 653–654 (1985).

15 Frasca, D.; Garavini, M.; Doria, G.: Recovery of T-cell function in aged mice injected with synthetic thymosin α-1. Cell. Immunol. *72:* 384–391 (1982).

16 Goya, R.; Sosa, Y.; Meites, J.: Half-life of plasma growth hormone in young and old conscious female rats. Exp. Gerontol. *22:* 27–36 (1987).

17 Grossman, A.; Stubbs, W.; Gaillard, R.; DeLitala, G.; Rees, L.; Besser, G.: Studies of the opiate control of prolactin, GH and TSH. Clin. Endocrin. *14:* 381–386 (1981).

18 Han, V.; D'Ercole, A.; Lund, P.: Cellular localization of somatomedin (insulin-like growth factor) messenger RNA in the human fetus. Science *236:* 193–197 (1987).

19 Ho, K.; Evans, W.; Blizzard, R.; Veldhuis, J.; Merriam, G.; Samojlik, E.; Furlanetto, R.; Rogol, A.; Kaiser, D.; Thorner, M.: Effects of sex and age on the 24-hour profile of growth hormone secretion in man: importance of endogenous estradiol concentrations. J. clin. Endocr. Metab. *64:* 51–58 (1987).

20 Huang, H.; Simpkins, J.; Meites, J.: Hypothalamic norepinephrine and dopamine turnover in ovariectomized old rats treated with gonadal steroids. APS Speciality Meeting, Michigan State University (East Lansing 1979).

21 Johanson, A.; Blizzard, R.: Low somatomedin-C levels in older men rise in response to growth hormone administration. Johns Hopkins med. J. *149:* 115–117 (1981).

22 Kahler, L.; Gliessman, P.; Craven, J.; Hill, J.; Critchlow, V.: Loss of enhanced nocturnal growth hormone secretion in aging rhesus monkeys. Endocrinology *119:* 1281–1284 (1986).

23 Kato, Y.; Dupre, J.; Beck, J.: Plasma growth hormone in the anesthetized rat: effects of dibutyral cyclic AMP, prostaglandin E, adrenergic agents, vasopressin, chlorpromazine, amphetamine, and *L*-Dopa. Endocrinology *93:* 135–146 (1973).

24 Kay, M.: Immunological aspects of aging: early changes in thymic activity. Mech. Age. Dev. *28:* 193–218 (1984).

25 Kelley, K.; Brief, S.; Westly, H.; Novakofski, J.; Bechtel, P.; Simon, J.; Walker, E.: GH_3 pituitary adenoma cells can reverse thymic aging in rats. Proc. natn. Acad. Sci. *83:* 5663–5667 (1986).

26 Lal, S.; Martin, J.; Dela Vega, C.: Comparison of the effects of apomorphine and L-dopa on serum growth hormone levels in normal men. Clin. Endocrin. *4:* 277–283 (1975).

27 Lal, S.; Nari, N.; Cervantes, P.; Pulman, J.; Guyda, H.: Effects of naloxone and levellorphan on serum prolactin concentrations and apomorphin-induced growth hormone secretion. Acta psychiat. scand. *59:* 173–176 (1979).

28 Laron, A.; Doron, M.; Arnikan, B.: Plasma growth hormone in men and women over 70 years of age. Med. Sports Physical Activ Aging *4:* 126–129 (1970).

29 Makinodan, T.; Kay, M.: Age influence on the immune system. Adv. Immunol. *29:* 287–330 (1980).

30 Martin, J.: Brain mechanisms for the integration of growth hormone secretion. Physiologist *22:* 23–28 (1979).

31 Martin, J.; Tolis, G.; Woods, I.; Guyda, H.: Failure of naloxone to influence physiological growth hormone and prolactin secretion. Brain Res. *168:* 210–216 (1979).

32 Meites, J.; Sonntag, W.: Hypothalamic hypophysiotropic hormones and neuroendocrine regulation: current views. Annu. Rev. Pharmacol. Toxicol. *21:* 295–341 (1981).

33 Mims, R.; Stein, R.; Bethune, J.: The effect of a single dose of *L*-Dopa on pituitary hormones in acromegaly, obesity, and in normal subjects. J. clin. Endocr. Metab. *37:* 34–42 (1973).
34 Morley, J.; Baranetsky, N.; Wingert, T.; Carlson, H.; Hershmann, J.; Melmed, S.; Levin, S.; Jamison, K.; Weitzman, R.; Chang, R.; Varrner, A.: Endocrine effects of naloxone induced opiate receptor blockade. J. clin. Endocr. Metab. *50:* 251–257 (1980).
35 Mueller, G.; Simpkins, J.; Meites, J.; Moore, K.: Differential effects of dopamine agonists and haloperidol on release of prolactin, thyroid stimulating hormone, growth hormone, and luteinizing hormone in rats. Neuroendocrinology *20:* 121–129 (1976).
36 Pluskal, M.; Moreyra, M.; Burini, R.; Young, V.: Protein synthesis studies in skeletal muscle of aging rats. I. Alterations in nitrogen composition and protein synthesis using a crude polyribosome and pH 5 enzyme system. J. Geront. *39:* 385–391 (1984).
37 Prinz, P.; Weitzmann, E.; Cunningham, G.; Karacan, I.: Plasma growth hormone during sleep in young and aged men. J. Geront. *38:* 519–524 (1983).
38 Richardson, A.: The relationship between aging and protein synthesis; in Florini, J., Handbook of biochemistry in aging, pp. 70–105 (CRC Press, Boca Raton 1981).
39 Richman, R.; Weiss, J.; Hochberg, Z.; Florini, J.: Regulation of growth hormone release; evidence against negative feedback in rat pituitary cells. Endocrinology *108:* 2287–2292 (1981).
40 Roth, J.; Kaeberle, M.; Grier, R.; Hooper, J.; Spiegel, H.; McAllister, H.: Improvement in clinical condition and thymus morphological features associated with growth hormone. Am. J. vet. Res. *45:* 1151–1155 (1984).
41 Rudman, D.; Katner, M.; Rogers, C.; Lubin, M.; Fleming, G.; Bain, R.: Impaired growth hormone secretion in the adult population. J. clin. Invest. *67:* 1261–1269 (1981).
42 Sassin, J.; Parker, D.; Mace, J.; Gotlin, R.; Johnson, L.; Rossman, L.: Human growth hormone release: relation to slow-wave sleep and sleep-waking cycles. Science *165:* 513–515 (1969).
43 Shaar, C.; Frederickson, R.; Dininger, N.; Jackson, L.: Enkephalin analogues and naloxone modulate the release of growth hormone and prolactin – evidence for regulation by an endogenous opioid peptide in the brain. Life Sci. *21:* 853–860 (1977).
44 Shibasaki, T.; Shizume, K.; Nakahara, M.; Masuda, A.; Jibiki, K.; Demura, H.; Wakabayashi, I.; Ling, N.: Age-related changes in plasma GH response of GHRF in man. J. clin. Endocr. Metab. *58:* 212–214 (1984).
45 Simpkins, J.; Mueller, G.; Huang, H.; Meites, J.: Evidence for depressed catecholamine and enhanced serotonin metabolism in aging male rats: possible relation to gonadotropin secretion. Endocrinology *100:* 1672–1679 (1977).
46 Sonntag, W.; Forman, L.; Miki, N.; Ramos, T.; Arimura, A.; Meites, J.: Effects of CNS active drugs and somatostatin antiserum on growth hormone release in young and old male rats. Neuroendocrinology *33:* 73–81 (1981).
47 Sonntag, W.; Forman, L.; Miki, N.; Trapp, J.; Gottschall, P.; Meites, J.: *L*-Dopa restores amplitude of growth hormone pulses in old male rats to that observed in young male rats. Neuroendocrinology *34:* 163–169 (1982).

48 Sonntag, W.; Gottschall, P.; Meites, J.: Increased secretion of somatostatin-28 from hypothalamic neurons of aged rats in vitro. Brain Res. *380:* 229–234 (1986).
49 Sonntag, W.; Gough, M.: Growth hormone releasing hormone induced release of growth hormone in aging male rats: dependence on pharmacological manipulation and endogenous somatostatin release. Neuroendocrinology (in press).
50 Sonntag, W.; Hylka, V.; Meites, J.: Impaired ability of old male rats to secrete growth hormone in vivo but not in vitro in response to hpGRF(1–44). Endocrinology *113:* 2305–2308 (1983).
51 Sonntag, W.; Hylka, V.; Meites, J.: Growth hormone restores protein synthesis in skeletal muscle of old male rats. J. Geront. *40:* 689–694 (1984).
52 Sonntag, W.; Steger, R.; Forman, L.; Meites, J.: Decreased pulsatile release of growth hormone in old male rats. Endocrinology *107:* 1875–1879 (1980).
53 Takahashi, S.; Gottschall, P.; Quigley, K.; Goya, R.; Meites, J.: Growth hormone secretory patterns in young, middle-aged, and old female rats. Neuroendocrinology *46:* 137–142 (1987).
54 Takahashi, Y.; Kipnis, D.; Daughaday, W.: Growth hormone secretion during sleep. J. clin. Invest. *47:* 2079–2083 (1968).
55 Tannenbaum, G.; Ling, N.; Brazeau, P.: Somatostatin-28 is longer acting and more selective than somatostatin-14 on pituitary and pancreatic hormone release. Endocrinology *111:* 101–108 (1982).
56 Tannenbaum, G.; Martin, J.: Evidence for an endogenous ultradian rhythm governing growth hormone secretion in the rat. Endocrinology *98:* 562–568 (1976).
57 Tannenbaum, G.; Panerai, A.; Frisen, H.: Failure of beta-endorphin antiserum, naloxone and naltrexone to alter physiological growth hormone and insulin secretion. Life Sci. *25:* 1983–1990 (1979).
58 Vijayan, E.; Krulich, L.; McCann, S.: Catecholaminergic regulation of TSH and growth hormone release in ovariectomized and ovariectomized steroid primed rats. Neuroendocrinology *26:* 174–180 (1978).
59 Wade, A.; Szewczuk, M.: Aging, idiotype, repertoire shifts, and compartmentalization of the mucosal-associated lymphoid system. Adv. Immunol. *36:* 143–188 (1984).
60 Wakabayashi, I.; Demura, R.; Miki, N.; Ohmura, E.; Miyoshi, H.; Shizume, K.: Failure of naloxone to influence plasma growth hormone, prolactin, and cortisol secretions induced by insulin hypoglycemia. J. clin. Endocr. Metab. *50:* 597–603 (1981).
61 Wehrenberg, W.; Ling, N.: Absence of an age-related change in the pituitary response to growth hormone releasing hormone in rats. Neuroendocrinology *37:* 463–466 (1983).
62 Weksler, M.: The immune system and the aging process in man. Proc. Soc. exp. Biol. Med. *165:* 200–205 (1980).
63 Weksler, M.; Innes, J.; Goldstein, G.: Immunological studies of aging. IV. The contribution of thymic involution to the immune deficiencies of aging mice and reversal with thymopoietin$_{32-36}$. J. exp. Med. *148:* 996–1006 (1978).

Dr. William E. Sonntag, Department of Physiology and Pharmacology,
Bowman Gray School of Medicine of Wake Forest University,
300 South Hawthorne Road, Winston-Salem, NC 27103 (USA)

Interdiscipl. Topics Geront., vol. 24, pp. 125–133 (Karger, Basel 1988)

Vasopressin and Aging[1]

Vratislav Zbuzek, Vlasta K. Zbuzek

Department of Anesthesiology, University of Medicine and Dentistry, New Jersey Medical School, Newark, N.J., USA

Introduction

Although several decades ago there were indications that antidiuretic hormone (vasopressin, VP) might be involved in the aging process [1, 2], this neuropeptide has not come under scrutiny in aging research until recently. This is somewhat surprising in view of its neurohormone, hypophysiotropic messenger, and neurotransmitter [3] roles in the regulation and preservation of some important homeostatic life processes.

Aging and VP in the Hypothalamic-Neurohypophyseal System

Hypothalamus

Considerable disagreement has been obtained from both the histochemical studies of age-related change in VP biosynthetic activity and the measurement of hypothalamic VP content by radioimmunoassay. The observed differences in hypothalamic VP content appear to result from a number of variables such as species, strain, individual variation, age, experimental paradigms and techniques of VP detection.

The VP content of rodent hypothalamus was found to be increased in old mice [4], or unchanged in middle-aged Long-Evans rats [5] and in

[1] This work was supported by NIA grant R01 AG02778. We are grateful to Dr. Berta Scharrer of Albert Einstein College of Medicine, Dr. Reginald M. Archibald of the Rockefeller University and Dr. John Katz of the University of Medicine and Dentistry of New Jersey, for their invaluable comments and critique. We thank Ms. Ladonna Levell for her aid in the preparation of the manuscript.

isolated supraoptic and paraventricular nuclei of old Fischer 344 rats [6]. Contrary to these findings, a lower hypothalamic VP content was reported in senile rats of three different strains [7–11].

Morphometric and ultrastructural studies, using nonspecific staining procedures for VP, reported that its biosynthetic activity was increased in aged mice [12], Wistar rats [13, 14], and postmortem-isolated hypothalamus of elderly humans [15–17], but unchanged in aged Sprague-Dawley rats [18–20]. On the other hand, other investigators using similar techniques reported decreased activity in aged rats of four different strains [2, 18, 21, 22]. However, some of these techniques do not necessarily reflect VP-synthesizing activity since several neuropeptides (e.g. dynorphin, Leu-enkephalin) are known to coexist in the magnocellular neurons of the supraoptic and paraventricular nuclei. Immunochemical studies with specific antibodies for VP and oxytocin (OT) showed a decreased number of VP- but not of OT-synthesizing neurons in the hypothalamus of aged monkeys [23] and mice [24].

Our recent experimental work demonstrated decreased incorporation of ^{3}H-arginine into hypothalamic VP and its slower axonal transport in the old male Fischer 344 rat [11], supporting the view that VP synthesis in aging is impaired, rather than enhanced, at least in the rat.

Neurohypophysis

There seems to be agreement that neurohypophyseal storage capacity is unaffected by aging. Several studies report an increased amount of neurosecretory material in middle-aged Wistar [25] and VP content of middle-aged Long-Evans [5], aged Sprague-Dawley [8] and Fischer 344 [9, 11, 26, 27] rats which, in fact, reflects the increasing size (weight) of the neurohypophysis with age. Other studies have reported that its content of VP did not change in aged rats [2, 6], mice [4] or human autopsy material [28]. Morphological and histochemical indices of VP storage capacity were found unchanged in aged mice [29] and rats [2] or decreased in aged rats [30, 31].

Since neurohypophysis weight increases with age, VP concentration expressed in milligrams per gland and milligrams per protein is also an important indicator of age-related change. However, some investigators report VP concentration per milligram neurohypophysis while others give it per milligram neurointermediate lobe. Because the weight of the intermediate lobe declines with age in some strains of rats, these are not equivalent denominators. Thus, if similar VP concentrations are found in young and old rats when expressed per milligram neurointermediate lobe [7–9], it indicates lower VP concentrations per milligram neurohypophysis in old rats [26, 27].

VP Release from the Neurohypophysis

Our data indicate a 6-hour delay in the transport of tritiated VP to the neurohypophysis of old males compared with young and adult Fischer 344 rats [11]. However, no difference was evident in neurohypophyseal specific activity of the three groups 24 h after injection of ^{3}H-arginine into cerebral ventricles, indicating a marked decrease in the release of the labelled VP from the neurohypophysis of aged rats. This agrees with previous studies in which VP release from isolated superfused neurohypophyses was decreased in 30-month-old male Fischer 344 rats [26, 27]. We have also shown that the VP content of aged rat neurohypophysis is 20–40% higher and its release 10–20% lower than in young rats. However, VP concentration (per milligram neurohypophysis) in old animals declines by 30% and VP release by 50–60%. In regard to middle-aged rats, VP release from the superfused hypothalamic-neurohypophyseal unit was higher in 13- to 17-month-old Long Evans rats [5] than in the young ones, which were found to show an unusually low response to depolarization with high potassium.

Plasma VP Concentration and Aging

Basal Plasma VP Concentration

Data reporting on age-related plasma VP concentration, obtained mainly in humans and rats, are also divergent. Plasma VP concentration in elderly humans was reported to be increased [32–35], unaltered [36–38] or decreased [39, 40]. Similarly, in aged rats, it was increased in Wistars [13, 32, 41], unaltered in Fischer 344 [6] or decreased in three different strains [8, 9, 42].

Responses to Physiological Stimuli

In response to dehydration, plasma VP levels were elevated [34, 37] or lowered [39] in elderly humans and in old Fischer 344 rats [6] in comparison with young subjects. In elderly humans, orthostatic hypotension failed to increase plasma VP [38], and alcohol-induced decline in plasma VP concentration was less marked [37].

The great variance in age-related changes in plasma VP concentration appears to result from a number of variables, some of which are mentioned above. The difficulty in distinguishing normal from pathological aspects of aging appears to be greater in human than in animal studies. Seasonal variations in plasma VP concentration, described in young subjects [43, 44] must also be considered.

VP Degradation

The only study done in a few elderly subjects under basal conditions [36] suggests that no age-related change occurs in the rate of disappearance of exogenous VP from the plasma. On the contrary, we recently demonstrated a higher VP clearance from liver of old Fischer 344 rats perfused in situ than from young and adult livers [45]. However, the rate of VP degradation in aged subjects exposed to various stimuli has not been studied.

Comparison of VP and OT in Aging

Recently, we have compared VP and OT levels in plasma and in hypothalamic-neurohypophyseal tissue, and their release from the isolated neurohypophysis in two strains of rats, to assess whether age-related differences are demonstrable. The data provide further evidence of impaired VP secretion under different experimental conditions.

Contrary to VP, plasma OT concentration and hypothalamic content were unaltered in aged Fischer 344 rats [46, and unpubl. data in collaboration with Fuchs]. Aging affected OT and VP release from the superfused neurohypophysis in a differential manner. Most striking was the difference in basal release (fig. 1). Basal OT release per gland was increased in aged Sprague-Dawley and Fischer 344 rats, whereas VP release was decreased in the former and did not change in the latter. Basal concentrations of released OT did not change whereas released VP decreased in aged rats of both strains under various experimental conditions.

Regulatory Mechanisms, VP and Aging

There is considerable evidence that VP secretion is centrally regulated by some classical neurotransmitters (acetylcholine, GABA, catecholamines) and a number of neuropeptides (angiotensin II, substance P, CRF,

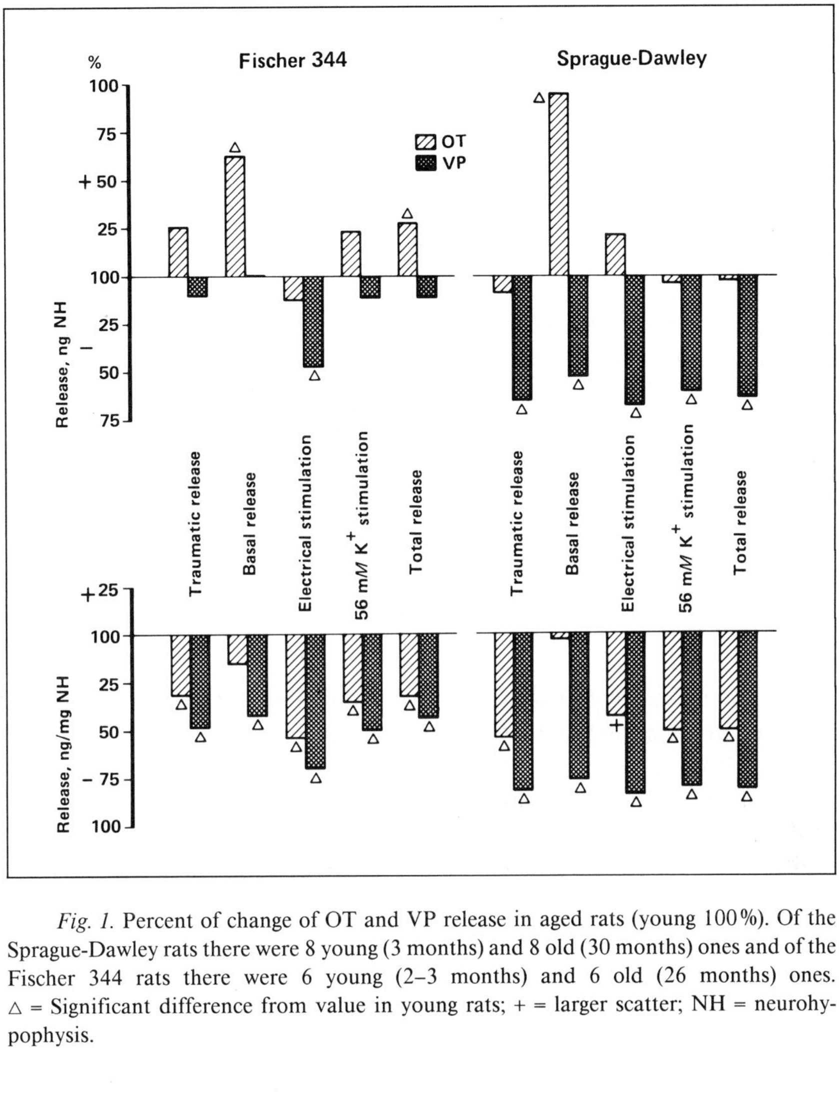

Fig. 1. Percent of change of OT and VP release in aged rats (young 100%). Of the Sprague-Dawley rats there were 8 young (3 months) and 8 old (30 months) ones and of the Fischer 344 rats there were 6 young (2–3 months) and 6 old (26 months) ones. △ = Significant difference from value in young rats; + = larger scatter; NH = neurohypophysis.

vasoactive intestinal polypeptide, and opioid peptides). Some means by which these regulators operate, themselves undergo age-related change. However, none of these regulators have been studied in respect to VP regulation during aging.

Recently, a negative-feedback endocrine loop was suggested to exist between VP and atrial natriuretic factor (ANF). VP appears to stimulate

ANF, which in turn was shown to suppress VP release [47]. A significant positive correlation with age was found in plasma ANF concentration in humans [48], implying that an ANF feedback mechanism may suppress VP release in older individuals. This, however, remains to be determined.

VP may affect certain behavioral and memory functions. Systematically administered VP apparently improved age-related deficit in conditioned avoidance behavior [49], prevented memory deficit, and enhanced cholinergic activity in rats [50].

Finally, our knowledge is only fragmentary of VP's involvement with the aging process in its neurotransmitter role. Recently, a marked age-related decrease was described in the density of VP- but not OT-containing fibers in a number of extrahypothalamic areas of rat brain [51]. This suggests that the neurotransmitter role of VP, but not of OT, may change as a function of age.

Conclusions

Is VP in the hypothalamic-neurohypophyseal pathway activated or inhibited in the aging process? This question has generated divergent views which still persist. Recent findings of decreased VP biosynthesis, transport, and rate of release considered with the many morphometric, cytochemical, ultrastructural, and biochemical observations of age-related change appear to support the view that the vasopressinergic system, at least in the rat, is specifically impaired in a nonparallel, differential manner to that of OT. A number of questions remain to be solved. For example, can rodent data apply to aging humans? Further studies are needed to explore the influence of regulatory mechanisms on VP under various conditions and to learn about its degradation in order to obtain a more accurate picture of the changes involved in VP secretion.

In addition to its antidiuretic activity, VP is now known to play an important role in homeostatic and integrative functions, behaving (1) as a neurotransmitter in neuronal communication pathways of the CNS, (2) as a hypophysiotropic messenger of the hypothalamic-anterior pituitary pathway, and (3) as an antagonist to ANF in the negative-feedback mechanism. However, it remains to be determined how these more recently discovered roles of VP relate to the aging process.

References

1 Findley, T.: Role of neurohypophysis in the pathogenesis of hypertension and some allied disorders associated with aging. Am. J. Med. *7:* 70–84 (1949).

2 Rodeck, H.; Lederis, K.; Heller, H.: The hypothalamo-neurohypophyseal system in old rats. J. Endocr. *21:* 225–230 (1960).

3 Scharrer, B.: Neurosecretion: beginnings and new directions in neuropeptide research. Annu. Rev. Neurosci. *10:* 1–17 (1987).

4 Rogers, J.; Shoemaker, W.J.; Morgan, D.G.; Finch, C.E.: Senescent change in tissue weight and immunoreactive β-endorphin, enkephalin, and vasopressin in eight regions of C57BL/6J mouse brain and pituitary. Neurobiol. Aging *6:* 1–9 (1985).

5 Miller, M.: Increased vasopressin secretion: an early manifestation of aging in the rat. J. Geront. *42:* 3–7 (1987).

6 Sladek, C.D.; McNeill, T.H.; Gregg, C.M.; Blair, M.L.; Baggs, R.B.: Vasopressin and renin response to dehydration in aged rats. Neurobiol. Aging *2:* 293–302 (1981).

7 Dorsa, D.M.; Bottemiller, L.: Age-related changes of vasopressin content of microdissected areas of the rat brain. Brain Res. *242:* 151–156 (1982).

8 Zbuzek, V.K.; Wu, W.: Age-related vasopressin changes in rat plasma and hypothalamo-hypophyseal system. Exp. Gerontol. *17:* 133–138 (1982).

9 Zbuzek, V.K.; Zbuzek, V.; Wu, W.: The effect of aging on vasopressin system in Fisher 344 rats. Exp. Gerontol. *18:* 395–311 (1983).

10 Landfield, P.W.; Sundberg, D.K.; Smith, M.S.; Eldridge, J.C.; Morris, M.: Mammalian aging: theoretical implications of changes in brain and endocrine systems during mid- and late-life in rats. Peptides *1,* suppl. 1, pp. 185–196 (1980).

11 Zbuzek, V.K.; Zbuzek, V.; Wu, W.: Age-related differences in the incorporation of ^{3}H-arginine into vasopressin in Fischer 344 rats. Exp. Gerontol. *22:* 113–125 (1987).

12 Davies, I.; Fotheringham,. A.P.: The influence of age on the hypothalamo-neurohypophyseal system of the mouse: a quantitative ultrastructural analysis of the supraoptic nucleus. Mech. Age. Dev. *12:* 93–105 (1980).

13 Fliers, E.; Swaab, D.F.: Activation of vasopressinergic and oxytocinergic neurons during aging in the Wistar rat. Peptides *4:* 165–170 (1983).

14 Kobayashi, Y.; Kawashima, S.; Arimatsu, Y.; Amano, T.: Binding of α-bungarotoxin to the supraoptic nucleus in male rats of various ages. Zool. Sci. *3:* 139–144 (1986).

15 Fliers, E.; Swaab, D.F.; Pool, C.W.; Verwer, R.W.H.: The vasopressin and oxytocin neurons in the human supraoptic and paraventricular nucleus; changes with aging and in senile dementia. Brain Res. *342:* 45–53 (1985).

16 Hoogendijk, J.E.; Fliers, E.; Swaab, D.F.; Verwer, R.W.H.: Activation of vasopressin neurons in the human supraoptic and paraventricular nucleus in senescence and senile dementia. J. neurol. Sci. *69:* 291–299 (1985).

17 Hommes, O.R.: Effects of hypophysectomy and age on the infundibular nucleus in man. J. Endocr. *62:* 479–488 (1974).

18 Kawashima, S.; Kobayashi, Y.: Morphometric study of the hypothalamo-neurohypophyseal system in aged rat. J. Sci. Hiroshima Univ. *30:* 229–242 (1982).

19 Peng, M.T.; Hsu, H.K.: No neuron loss from hypothalamic nuclei of old male rats. Gerontology *28:* 19–22 (1982).

20 Hsu, H.K.; Peng, M.T.: Hypothalamic neuron number of old female rats. Gerontology *24:* 434–440 (1978).
21 Lin, K.H.; Peng, Y.M.; Peng, M.T.; Tseng, T.M.: Changes in the nuclear volume of rat hypothalamic neurons in old age. Neuroendocrinology *21:* 247–254 (1976).
22 Watkins, W.B.; Choy, V.J.: The impact of aging on neuronal morphology in rat hypothalamo-neurohypophysial system: an immunohistochemical study. Peptides *1:* suppl. 1, pp. 239–245 (1980).
23 Sladek, J.R.; McConnel, J.; McNeill,T.H.: Integrated morphology of neuronal catecholamines and neurophysin in the aged macaque. Adv. exp. Med. Biol. *113:* 241–250 (1978).
24 Kawamoto, K.; Kawashima, S.: Changes of vasopressin- and oxytocin-immunoreactive neurons after hypophysectomy in young and old mice. Exp. Gerontol. *20:* 295–304 (1985).
25 Morrison, A.B.; Staroscik, R.N.: The neurosecretory substance in the neurohypophysis of the rat during maturation and aging. Gerontologia *9:* 65–70 (1964).
26 Zbuzek, V.; Zbuzek, V.K.; Wu, W.: Vasopressin release from individually superfused neurohypophyses decreases in aged rats. Neuroendocrinology *39:* 538–548 (1984).
27 Zbuzek, V.K.; Zbuzek, V.; Wu, W.: Decremental vasopressin release after repeated stimulation of superfused neurohypophyses of Fisher 344 rats of different ages. J. Geront. *41:* 140–146 (1986).
28 Currier, A.R.; Adamson, H.; Dyke, H.B. van: Vasopressin and oxytocin in the posterior lobe of the pituitary of man. J. clin. Endocr. Metab. *20:* 947–951 (1960).
29 Wilkinson, A.; Davies, I.: The influence of age on the hypothalamo-neurohypophyseal system of mouse: a quantitative ultrastructural analysis of the posterior pituitary. Mech. Age. Dev. *15:* 129–139 (1981).
30 Dunihue, F.W.: Reduced juxtaglomerular cell granularity, pituitary neurosecretory material, and width of the zona glomerulosa in aging rats. Endocrinology *77:* 948–951 (1965).
31 Rechardt, L.; Hervonen, H.: Ultrastructural changes in the neurohypophysis of the aged male rat. Cell Tiss. Res. *226:* 51–62 (1982).
32 Frolkis, V.V.; Golovchenko, S.F.; Medvedev, V.I.; Frolkis, R.A.: Vasopressin and cardiovascular system in aging. Gerontology *28:* 290–302 (1982).
33 Kirkland, J.; Lye, M.; Goddard, C.; Vargas, E.; Davies, I.: Plasma arginine vasopressin in dehydrated elderly patients. Clin. Endocrinol. *20:* 451–456 (1984).
34 Phillips, P.A.; Rolls, B.J.; Ledingham, J.G.G.; Forsling, M.L.; Morton, J.J.; Crowe, M.J.; Wollner, L.: Reduced thirst after water deprivation in healthy elderly men. New Engl. J. Med. *311:* 753–759 (1984).
35 Os, I.; Kjeldsen, S.E.; Aakesson, I.; Skjoto, J.; Eide, I.; Hjermann, I.; Leren, P.: Evidence of age-related variation in plasma vasopressin of normotensive men. Scand. J. clin. Lab. Invest. *45:* 263–268 (1985).
36 Engel, P.A.; Rowe, J.W.; Minaker, K.L.; Robertson, G.L.: Effect of exogenous vasopressin on vasopressin release. Am. J. Physiol. *246:* E202–E207 (1984).
37 Helderman, J.H.; Vestal, R.E.; Rowe, J.W.; Tobin, J.D.; Andres, R.; Robertson, G.L.: The response of arginine vasopressin to intravenous ethanol and hypertonic saline in man: the impact of aging. J. Geront. *33:* 39–47 (1978).

38 Rowe, J.W.; Minaker, K.L.; Sparrow, D.; Robertson, G.L.: Age-related failure of volume-pressure-mediated vasopressin release. J. clin. Endocr. Metab. *54:* 661–664 (1982).
39 Li, C.H.; Hsieh, S.M.; Nagai, I.: The response of plasma arginine vasopressin to 14 h water deprivation in the elderly. Acta endocr. *105:* 314–317 (1984).
40 Kendler, K.S.; Weitzman, R.E.; Fisher, D.A.: The effect of pain on plasma arginine vasopressin concentrations in man. Clin. Endocrinol. *8:* 89–94 (1978).
41 Kobayashi, Y.; Lederis, K.; Kawashima, S.: Neural lobe function in aged Wistar/Tw strain rats showing polydipsia and polyuria. Endocr. jap. *33:* 617–627 (1986).
42 Turkington, M.R.; Everitt, A.V.: The neurohypophysis and aging with special reference to the antidiuretic hormone; in Everitt, Burgess, Hypothalamus, pituitary and aging, p. 123 (Thomas, Springfield 1976).
43 MacFarlane, W.V.; Robinson, K.W.: Seasonal changes in plasma antidiuretic activity produced by a standard heat stimulus. J. Physiol. *135:* 1–11 (1957).
44 Zbuzek, V.K.; Wu, W.: Seasonal variations in vasopressin secretion in rats. Experientia *35:* 1523–1524 (1979).
45 Shih, A.P.; Zbuzek, V.K.; Sauchelli, F.C.; Wu, W.: Aging and vasopressin degradation (Abstract). J. clin. Pharm. *25:* 467 (1985).
46 Zbuzek, V.; Fuchs, A.R.; Zbuzek, V.K.; Wu, W.: Age- and strain-related differences in vasopressin and oxytocin release (Abstract No. 315). 1st Int. Cong. Neuroendocrinol., San Francisco 1986.
47 Manning, P.T.; Schwartz, D.; Katsube, N.C.; Holmberg, S.W.; Needleman, P.: Vasopressin-stimulated release of atriopeptin: endocrine antagonists in fluid homeostasis. Science *229:* 395–397 (1985).
48 Larochelle, P.; Cusson, J.R.; Gutkowska, J.; Schiffrin, E.L.; Hamet, P.; Kuchel, O.; Genest, J.; Cantin, M.: Plasma atrial natriuretic factor concentrations in essential and renovascular hypertension. Br. med. J. *294:* 1249–1252 (1987).
49 Cooper, R.L.; McNamara, M.C.; Thompson, W.G.: Vasopressin and conditioned flavor aversion in aged rats. Neurobiol. Aging *1:* 53–57 (1980).
50 Meck, W.H.; Church, R.M.; Wenk, G.L.: Arginine vasopressin innoculates against age-related increases in sodium-dependent high affinity choline uptake and discrepancies in the content of temporal memory. Eur. J. Pharmacol. *130:* 327–331 (1986).
51 Fliers, E.; Vries, G.J. de; Swaab, D.F.: Changes with aging in the vasopressin and oxytocin innervation of rat brain. Brain Res. *348:* 1–8 (1985).

V. Zbuzek, PhD, Department of Anesthesiology, UMD-New Jersey Medical School, 185 South Orange Avenue, Newark, NJ 07103–2757 (USA)

Interdiscipl. Topics Geront., vol. 24, pp. 134–140 (Karger, Basel 1988)

Rejuvenation of Sexual Behavior of Aging Rats with Neurotransmitters

M.T. Peng[a], *F.J. Yang*[a], *S.C. Mu*[a], *H.K. Hsu*[b], *P.S. Wang*[c], *S.Y. Lue*[d]

[a] Departments of Physiology, College of Medicine, National Taiwan University,
[b] Kaohsiung Medical College, [c] National Yangming Medical College, and
[d] General Triservice Hospital, Taipei, Taiwan

Introduction

As age advances, copulatory activity of male rats declines remarkably [7, 8, 10] but the lordosis response – assumption of the normal female copulatory position – decreases only in some female rats [1, 14]. Age-related changes in brain neurotransmitter activity or receptors have been observed [16–19, 22] and it has been reported that hyperprolactinemia [21], endorphin, serotonin (5-HT) and noradrenaline (NA) inhibit copulatory activity of young adult male rats [3, 5] whereas dopamine (DA) enhances it. Also, prolactin, NA and DA inhibit the lordosis response of young adult female rats [3, 5]. These findings suggest that pharmacological intervention can be used to improve or rejuvenate age-related changes in sexual behavior.

Neurotransmitter agonists and antagonists, which have been reported to enhance sexual behavior in adult rats, were tested in older rats to learn whether they could improve their lowered sexual activity and to elucidate the causal relationship between sexual behavior in old age and changes in brain content of neurotransmitters.

Gonadectomized Rats with Testosterone or Estradiol Replacement

Long-Evans rats, both male and female, 2 years or older, were gonadectomized and immediately implanted subcutaneously with a hormone-filled Silastic capsule. Males received testosterone in capsules measuring

80 mm length with 1.57 mm internal diameter and 3.18 mm outside diameter and females were given estradiol benzoate (EB):cholesterol (1:1) in capsules measuring 1 mm/100 g body weight.

Prior to pharmacological treatment, all old male rats showed low copulatory activity. Only old female rats which showed a lordosis quotient (LQ) below 50 were selected for treatment. Sexual behavior was monitored in the same animals before and after drug treatment.

Copulatory Activity

Pharmacological treatment did not obviously improve sexual activity in old male rats, which did not display any mount, intromission and ejaculation prior to drug treatment. In the rats which showed some mount and intromission but no ejaculation, apomorphine *p*-chlorophenylalanine (PCPA), and methysergide improved the frequency of mount and intromission but bromocriptine, *L*-dopa and naloxone were ineffec-

Table I. Effects of neurotransmitter agonists and antagonists on the copulatory activity of old male rats which showed mounting and intromission but no ejaculation

Rats n	Age months	Drug treatment		Mount frequency[1]	Intromission frequency	Ejaculation frequency
9	24.9 ± 1.8	apomorphine	before	10.7 ± 1.3	19.9 ± 3.4	0
		20 mg/kg (sc)	after	16.9 ± 2.5**	19.5 ± 1.0	2 (2)
8	28.5 ± 1.7	bromocriptine	before	9.0 ± 2.4	10.0 ± 2.7	0
		4 mg/kg/day × 10 days (sc)	after	9.7 ± 3.1	9.0 ± 2.6	0
7	22.1 ± 1.1	*L*-dopa (sc)	before	11.3 ± 2.9	15.5 ± 7.5	0
		100 mg/kg twice daily × 10	after	14.0 ± 4.9	16.0 ± 7.3	1 (1)
9	25.1 ± 1.9	naloxone	before	10.9 ± 1.9	14.2 ± 4.6	0
		4 mg/kg (ip)	after	10.1 ± 1.0	15.2 ± 2.6	1 (3)
7	27.2 ± 1.4	PCPA	before	14.1 ± 2.9	18.0 ± 3.6	0
		150 mg/kg (ip)	after	23.9 ± 3.0**	23.0 ± 3.9**	1 (1)
7	27.9 ± 0.9	methysergide	before	13.6 ± 1.8	15.1 ± 2.9	0
		3 mg/kg (ip)	after	16.9 ± 2.6*	24.1 ± 4.5*	0

Mean ± SEM. The figures in parentheses indicate number of rats showing ejaculation. * 5 %, ** 1 %, significant difference versus pretreatment.

[1] Parameters of copulatory activity during 30-min test.

tive (table I). The result is consistent with the enhancing effect of PCPA on poor copulators [12] and the activation of estrous behavior in adult female rats [13]. Few rats ejaculated after the injection of all drugs (table I) and neither mount latency nor intromission latency changed significantly. Since apomorphine (a DA receptor stimulant), PCPA (an inhibitor of 5-HT synthesis), and methysergide (a 5-HT receptor blocker) improved copulatory activity of old rats, combinations of apomorphine and PCPA or methysergide were tried to see if they produced a synergistic effect. When combined, to our surprise, the apomorphine cancelled out the improvement on copulatory activity induced by PCPA or by methysergide.

PCPA has been reported to diminish the effectiveness of *L*-dopa in reestablishing luteinizing hormone surge in old constant-estrus rats [23]. Besides stimulating DA receptors, apomorphine increases 5-HT content in the dorsal raphe cell bodies and in the striatum [11], which would antagonize the 5-HT depleting action of PCPA. In addition to this effect, PCPA decreases brain DA and NA [15], which would antagonize the DA receptor-stimulating action of apomorphine. Methysergide also has DA agonist-antagonist activity [2].

Naloxone has been reported to be able to improve copulatory activity in sexually inactive rats. However, in the present study it did not effectively improve sexual behavior in old rats. Naloxone has reduced ability in old rats to stimulate luteinizing hormone and testosterone release [20]. Dorsa et al. [4] and Steger et al. [20] have suggested that the reduced response of old rats to naloxone may be due to high endogenous levels or high turnover rates of brain opioids. Increased Met-enkephalin content in the hypothalamus was observed in old male rats [20], but not in old female rats [9]. Another possibility of reduced response of old rats to naloxone is that they have fewer opioid receptors. Decreased concentrations of opioid receptors were found in the hypothalamus and other brain regions of aged rats [16]. From this evidence, the inability of naloxone to improve sexual behavior of old rats does not seem to contradict the results of Dorsa et al. [4]. Serum testosterone concentration was 5.49 $\pm$ 0.38 ng/ml (n = 10).

Diminished levels of β-endorphin were found in the hypothalamus of old male rats, especially in the behaviorally inactive subgroup [4]. From this result, Dorsa et al. [4] suspected that β-endorphin might be secreted in greater quantities in the sexually active group than in the age-matched but sexually inactive group.

Table II. Effects of neurotransmitter agonists and antagonists on the lordosis response of old female rats which showed low receptivity

Drugs		Rats n	Age months	LQ pre-treatment	LQ post-treatment
Bromocriptine	(4 mg/kg/day × 10 days)	9	25.7±0.5	15.6±7.5	22.2±12.6
Naloxone	(4 mg/kg ip)	9	27.5±1.4	8.9±4.0	16.1±10.0
AMPT	(100 mg/kg ip)	10	26.7±1.5	20.9±4.2	39.7±14.3
PCPA	100 mg/kg/day × 4 days	21	28.5±0.8	16.9±3.8	52.1±5.9**
	20 mg/kg/day × 4 days	11	28.5±0.2	17.7±6.7	43.6±9.9*
Methysergide	(3 mg/kg ip)	11	26.7±0.1	15.5±5.5	55.5±9.3**

Mean ± SEM. * 5 %; ** 1 %; significant difference versus pretreatment.

Lordosis Quotient

Eighty-eight old female rats were tested. Among them 40 rats showed prolonged vaginal cornification more than 2 weeks before ovariectomy, 42 showed irregular cycles, and 6 were pseudopregnant (PSP) prior to ovary removal. The response of prolonged-vaginal-cornification rats and cyclic rats to drugs did not differ so their results are pooled. As shown in table II, PCPA and methysergide improved the LQ, but α-methyl-*p*-tyrosine (AMPT), bromocriptine and naloxone could not. Among 6 PSP rats, LQ improved in 1 rat treated with AMPT, in 1 rat treated with methysergide, and 1 out of 2 each treated with PCPA and naloxone. Although the number of PSP rats is not large enough, the data suggest that these neurotransmitter agonists and antagonists can also improve receptivity of PSP rats. Solicitation behavior was displayed so infrequently that the measure was dropped from analysis.

Brain monoamine levels of young and old ovariectomized rats with EB replacement were measured by high-performance liquid chromatography with electrochemical detection and were compared with those of similarly treated old female rats after PCPA injection. Old rats had higher levels of 5-HT in the preoptic area (POA) plus hypothalamus than did young rats ($p < 0.01$). This is consistent with the findings of Timiras et al. [22].

PCPA reduced 5-HT and 5-HIAA level in POA plus hypothalamus tissue to 26% when given for 4 days at the dose of 100 mg/kg/day (ta-

Table III. Effects of PCPA on the level of 5-HT and its metabolite 5-HIAA in the brain of old female rats treated with estradiol

	Young (n = 8)	Old (n = 7)	Old + PCPA 100 mg/kg (n = 11)	Old + PCPA 20 mg/kg (n = 10)
Hypothalamus plus POA				
5-HT	797.5±129.3	1,339.2±243.7*	207.5±33.2**	1,224.3±50.1
5-HIAA	1,086.2±102.9	1,427.5±280.1	174.0±24.2**	856.9±72.7
5-HIAA/5-HT	1.20±0.08	1.06±0.05	1.00±0.18	0.69±0.05
Remaining brain				
5-HT	726.9±63.7	990.0±201.5	177.8±25.7**	
5-HIAA	2,620.9±318.8	3,362.3±612.0	443.9±61.0	
5-HIAA/5-HT	3.56±0.34	3.86±0.63	2.87±0.37	

Mean ± SEM. The values are given as nanograms per gram wet weight, the doses of PCPA as milligrams per kilogram per day for 4 days. * 5%; ** 1%, significant difference versus young rats.

ble III). Therefore, the improvement caused by this dose seems to be pharmacological. At the dose of 20 mg/kg/day over a 4-day period, PCPA increased the lordosis response but 5-HT and 5-HIAA levels of the POA plus hypothalamus did not change although the 5-HIAA/5-HT ratio was lower than that of young and old rats without PCPA treatment. These results suggest that high brain levels of 5-HT or elevation of its turnover rate play a crucial role in the lowered lordotic response characteristic of old rats.

Hyperprolactinemia was observed in old female rats, the values being 354 ± 39 ng/ml (n = 7) compared to 122± 28 ng/ml (n = 7) in young females. This condition was not seen in old male rats which had prolactin levels of 55 ± 8 ng/ml (n = 8). Bromocriptine decreased elevated serum prolactin levels of old female rats to the level of young rats (141 ± 37 ng/ml) (n = 8), but could not improve receptivity of old female rats. Apparently, hyperprolactinemia does not play a critical role in decreased sexual behavior of old female rats. *L*-Dopa and bromocriptine depressed serum prolactin levels of old male rats below normal levels to 19 ± 4 ng/ml (n = 13) and 4 ng/ml (n = 2), respectively, but did not increase their copulatory activity.

Ovariectomized Rats with EB plus Progesterone Treatment

Ovariectomized rats were injected subcutaneously with a dose of 0.3 ng/100 g/day EB for 2 days. On the 3rd day, the rats were injected subcutaneously with 0.5 mg progesterone about 1 h before the lights were turned off. Receptivity testing began 4–6 h after progesterone injection. The improvement in lordosis quotient after PCPA was 15.7 ± 6.9 (before) versus 41.4 ± 11.6 (after) with $p < 0.05$ (n = 7) and for methysergide it was 34.4 ± 4.7 (before) versus 56.7 ± 7.8 (after) with $p < 0.05$ (n = 9).

Conclusions

PCPA and methysergide were the neurotransmitter antagonists most capable of improving copulatory activity in castrated old male rats treated with testosterone and in increasing the lordosis response of ovariectomized old female rats treated with EB alone or EB plus progesterone. Apomorphine also improved copulatory activity of old, castrated, testosterone-treated rats. Bromocriptine, *L*-dopa, naloxone, and AMPT were not effective. These results together with the data of brain monoamine levels indicate that increased brain serotonin activity and reduced dopamine uptake play a crucial role in decreased copulatory activity in old male rats. Elevated serotonin diminishes the lordosis response but hyperprolactinemia does not seem to be a critical factor in the decreased sexual behavior of old female rats.

References

1 Cooper, R.L.; Linnoila, M.: Sexual behavior in aged noncyclic female rats. Physiol. Behav. *18:* 573–576 (1977).
2 Creese, I.; Burt, D.R.; Snyder, S.H.: The dopamine receptor: differential binding of α-LSD and related agents to agonist and antagonist states. Life Sci. *17:* 1715–1719 (1975).
3 Crowley, W.R.; Zemlan, F.P.: The neurochemical control of mating behavior; in Adler, Neuroendocrinology of reproduction, pp. 451–484 (Plenum Press, New York 1981).
4 Dorsa, D.M.; Smith, E.R.; Davidson, J.M.: Immunoreactive β-endorphin and LHRH levels in the brains of aged male rats with impaired sex behavior. Neurobiol. Aging *5:* 115–120 (1984).
5 Dudley, C.A.; Jamison, T.S.; Moss, R.L.: Inhibition of lordosis behavior in the female rat by intraventricular infusion of prolactin. Endocrinology *110:* 677–679 (1982).

6 Gessa, G.L.; Pagliette, E.: Induction of copulatory behavior in sexually inactive rats by naloxone. Science *204:* 203–205 (1979).
7 Gray, G.D.; Smith, E.R.; Dorsa, D.M.; Davidson, J.M.: Sexual behavior and testosterone in middle-aged male rats. Endocrinology *109:* 1597–1604 (1981).
8 Hsu, H.K.; Hsu, C.; Yu, J.Y.L.; Peng, M.T.: Effects of long-term testosterone replacement on copulatory activity in old male rats. Gerontology *32:* 10–17 (1986).
9 Kumar, M.S.A.; Chen, C.L.; Huang, H.H.: Pituitary and hypothalamic concentration of Met-enkephalin in young and old rats. Neurobiol. Aging *1:* 153–155 (1980).
10 Larsson, K.: Sexual activity in senile male rats. Gerontology *13:* 136–139 (1958).
11 Lee, E.H.Y.; Geyer, M.A.: Selective effects of apomorphine on dorsal raphe neurons: a cytofluorimetric study. Brain Res. Bull. *9:* 719–725 (1982).
12 Malmnas, C.O.; Meyerson, B.J.: *p*-Chlorophenylalanine facilitates copulatory behavior in male rats. Nature *232:* 398–401 (1971).
13 Meyerson, B.J.; Lewander, T.: Serotonin synthesis inhibition and estrous behavior in female rats. Life Sci. *9:* 661–671 (1970).
14 Peng, M.T.; Chuong, C.F.; Peng, Y.M.: Lordosis response of senile female rats. Neuroendocrinology *24:* 317–324 (1977).
15 Peters, D.A.; Filczewski, V.M.; Mazurkiewiez-Kwilecki, I.M.: Effect of para-chlorophenylalanine on catecholamine synthesis in rat brain, heart and adrenals. Biochem. Pharmac. *21:* 2282–2284 (1972).
16 Roth, G.S.: Brain dopaminergic and opiate receptors and responsiveness during aging; in Agnoli, Crepaldi, Spano, Trabucchi, Aging, vol. 23: Aging brain and ergot alkaloids, pp. 53–60 (Raven Press, New York 1983).
17 Severson, J.A.; Finch, C.E.: Reduced dopaminergic binding during aging in rodent striatum. Brain Res. *192:* 147–162 (1980).
18 Simpkins, J.W.; Mueller, G.P.; Huang, H.H.; Meites, J.: Evidence for depressed catecholamine and enhanced serotonin metabolism in aging male rats: possible relation to gonadotropin secretion. Endocrinology *100:* 1672–1678 (1977).
19 Simpkins, J.W.: Regional changes in monoamine metabolism in the aging constant estrous rat. Neurobiol. Aging. *5:* 309–313 (1984).
20 Steger, R.W.; Sonntag, W.E.; Van Nugt, D.A.; Forman, L.J.; Meites, J.: Reduced ability of naloxone to stimulate LH and testosterone release in aging male rats: possible relation to increase in hypothalamic Met-enkephalin. Life Sci. *27:* 747–753 (1980).
21 Svare, B.; Bartke, A.; Doherty, P.; Mason, I.; Michael, S.D.; Smith, M.S.: Hyperprolactinemia suppresses copulatory behavior in male rats and mice. Biol. Reprod. *21:* 529–535 (1979).
22 Timiras, P.S.; Hudson, D.B.; Segall, P.E.: Lifetime brain serotonin: regional effects of age and precursor availability. Neurobiol. Aging *5:* 235–242 (1984).
23 Walker, R.F.: Reinstatement of LH surges by serotonin neuroleptics in aging constant estrous rats. Neurobiol. Aging *3:* 253–257 (1982).

Prof. M.T. Peng, Department of Physiology, National Taiwan University,
No 1 Jen Al Road, 1st Section, Taipei (Taiwan)

Interdiscipl. Topics Geront., vol. 24, pp. 141–149 (Karger, Basel 1988)

Rejuvenation of the Aging Hypothalamic-Pituitary Axis with Fetal Hypothalamic Graft[1]

Henry H. Huang.

Department of Research, Mercy Hospital and Medical Center, Chicago, Ill., USA

Introduction

One of the most characteristic events of aging in many mammalian species is a gradual decline in reproductive function. Rats exhibit a gradual reduction in sexual activity and fertility with increase in age [1, 2]. Based on many previous studies, we and many other investigators believe that the decline of neuroendocrine and reproductive function in aging rodents may largely be attributed to the alteration of hypothalamic function. Lower activities of catecholamines and luteinizing-hormone-releasing hormone (LHRH) and a higher activity of serotonin in the hypothalamus of old rodents had been reported by our laboratory and others [3–5]. The decreased activities of catecholamines and LHRH in the hypothalamus of old rats may partly be due to the loss of hypothalamic neurons during aging [6, 7]. The neuroendocrine and reproductive function in old rats can be increased by injections of LHRH or catecholamine precursor, *L*-dopa [8, 9]. However, this acute administration of drugs only prompts acute stimulation of neuroendocrine and reproductive function. The neuroendocrine and reproductive function resumed to original status after ceasing the treatment. Our major interest is to find a more physiological and long-lasting approach to rejuvenate the hypothalamic-pituitary system in old age. Recently, some studies have shown that neural tissue from the CNS of fetal and neonatal mammals can survive, differentiate and function in a

[1] This study was supported by Grant AGO4351, awarded by the National Institute on Aging, NIH, Bethesda, MD 20205.

recipient brain of aged rodents [10–12]. The overall purpose of the present research is to attempt to use the fetal hypothalamic transplant to correct neuroendocrine deficiencies in senescent rats.

Methods

Fetal Hypothalamic Transplantation

Timed, pregnant, Long-Evans rats were deeply anesthetized by subcutaneous injection of 20 mg/kg sodium pentobarbital at 17–19 days of gestation. The fetuses were removed from the mother and sexed. The fetal brain was excised. The anterior hypothalamus was bisected and a block of tissue was dissected. An anterior cut 1.50 mm wide was made at the midline of the ventral side of the fetal brain just caudal to the bifurcation of the anterior cerebral artery; a second cut was made just caudal to the median eminence. A lateral cut was made 0.75 mm from the midline and the tissue block was finally cut 1.0 mm deep. It contained the developing preoptic area, supraoptic, suprachiasmatic, paraventricular and arcuate nuclei and median eminence. The tissue was then placed in a drop of sterile saline in a well slide on a bed of ice and bisected with a sharp microforcep. For each graft, a tissue block was cut as small as possible and drawn into a 20-gauge needle affixed to a stereotaxic instrument. The aged rat was anesthetized with 50 mg/kg ketamine HCl and inhalation of Penthrane during surgery. The needle of the syringe containing the transplant tissue was taken down in the midline of the brain into the third ventricle, just anterior-dorsal to the median eminence. Downward movement of the needle stylet deposited the tissue on to the median eminence. Controls were either without surgery or grafted with the same amount of cerebral cortex. The fetal hypothalamus was transplanted into the brain of aged hosts of same sex.

Brain Histology of Hypothalamic Transplant

Three months after fetal hypothalamic transplantation, the animals were sacrificed. Each brain was quickly removed and frozen with dry ice. The brain was sectioned at 30 μm thickness with every 10th section stained with cresyl violet in order to verify survival and anatomical orientation of the transplant. Only hosts with viable grafts were included in this study. Histological examination showed that well-vascularized hypothalamic grafts were growing in the third ventricle of host brains (fig. 1). This indicated that the grafted tissue was nourished by the blood of host brain. The third ventricle of host brain was enlarged and filled with viable transplants.

Results

Restoration of Sexual Function and Fertility by Fetal Hypothalamic Transplant in Impotent Aged Male Rats

Long-Evans male rats were born and raised in our laboratory. For testing sexual function, each male rat that reached 18–20 months of age was put overnight into a cage which contained 4 10- to 12-week-old

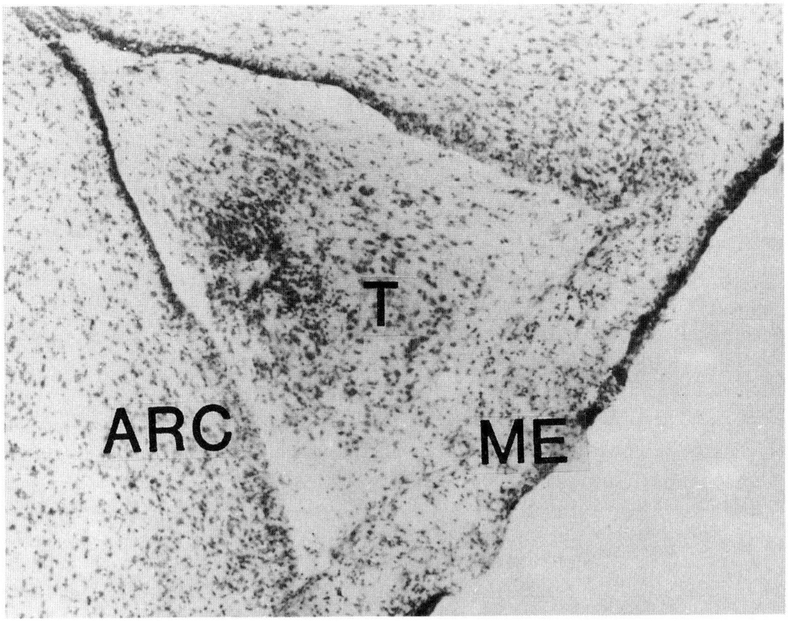

Fig. 1. Fetal anterior hypothalamic transplant in the third ventricle of aged impotent male rats. Low-power micrograph of a 30-μm coronal section, showing a transplant (T) filling and expanding the third ventricle. The base of the transplant is in apposition to the median eminence (ME) and arcuate nucleus (ARC) [from 19]. Cresyl violet. × 50.

females at proestrous stage. A vaginal smear of each female was monitored early the next morning. Sperm seen in the vaginal smear was regarded as copulation and ejaculation. For testing fertility, each female which copulated with an aged male was housed individually until the birth of the pups. The male rat which was not able to inseminate and impregnate females was regarded as impotent. The test was repeated twice, 1 week apart, and the higher score represented the sexual function and fertility of the males. The testing procedure was undertaken before and 1–2 months after fetal hypothalamic transplantation.

The effect of fetal hypothalamic transplant on the sexual function and fertility in impotent aged male rats is shown in table I. Seven out of ten hypothalamus-grafted males were restored to their sexual function and fertility. Three males ejaculated twice, 4 ejaculated once, resulting in the

Table I. Effect of fetal hypothalamic transplant on the sexual function and fertility of impotent aged male rats

Group and number of animals	Ejaculations		Number of females impregnated	
	number of animals	number/ animal/night[1]	before transplantation	after transplantation
Hypothalamus	3	2	0 (0)	9 (106)
graft (n = 10)	4	1		
	3	0		
Controls				
Untreated (n = 7)	7	0	0 (0)	0 (0)
Brain cortex graft (n = 4)	1	1	0 (0)	0 (0)
	3	0		

The figures in parentheses indicate the total number of pups born.
[1] One to two months after transplantation.

impregnation of 9 females and the fathering of 106 pups. The remaining 3 males did not respond to the transplantation. None of 7 untreated controls ejaculated and only 1 out of 4 males with a cerebral cortex graft ejaculated once, impregnating 1 female which delivered 6 pups.

Increased Secretion of Luteinizing Hormone and Testosterone by Fetal Hypothalamic Transplant in Impotent Aged Male Rats

Just before and 3 months after fetal hypothalamic transplantation, blood samples were taken by orbital sinus puncture under light ether anesthesia for measurements of luteinizing hormone (LH) and testosterone. At the end of experiment, the hypothalamic grafted old animals were sacrificed and the pituitary glands were removed for determination of pituitary LH.

Males with successful hypothalamic graft had significantly higher concentrations of pituitary LH than those of controls (1.52 ± 0.08 vs. 0.49 ± 0.08 and 0.91 ± 0.2 µg/mg protein; $p < 0.05$). Before transplantation the levels of serum LH were not significantly different between animals with hypothalamic grafts and controls. Two to three months after transplantation, a significant increase in serum LH was found in the males with successful hypothalamic grafts. The values rose from 0.68 ± 0.13 to $0.98 \pm$

0.09 ng/ml, $p < 0.05$. However, serum LH was significantly reduced in the untreated and cerebral-cortex-grafted animals. It declined from 0.76 ± 0.16 to 0.45 ± 0.07 ng/ml, $p < 0.05$, in untreated males and from 0.67 ± 0.10 to 0.44 ± 0.08 ng/ml, $p < 0.05$, in cortex-grafted controls. Similarly, males with successful hypothalamic grafts showed a significant increase in serum testosterone as compared to those before transplantation. It rose from 0.29 ± 0.04 to 1.04 ± 0.16 ng/ml, $p < 0.05$. Compared to pretransplantation values, serum testosterone was significantly decreased in both groups of controls. It fell from 0.67 ± 0.26 to 0.24 ± 0.07 ng/ml, $p < 0.05$, in untreated males, and from 0.76 ± 0.20 to 0.35 ± 0.08 ng/ml, $p < 0.05$, in cortex-transplanted controls. The decrease in serum LH and testosterone 3 months after transplantation in the untreated or cortex-transplanted controls could be due to the natural decline of gonadotropins and testosterone during aging process. The males with unsuccessful hypothalamic transplant were similar to those of controls. These indicate that the fetal hypothalamic tissue probably did not affect the brain of this group of aged hosts.

Effects of Fetal Hypothalamic Transplant on the Ovarian Function and Vaginal Cyclicity in Old Constant-Estrus Female Rats

In a pilot study, Matsumoto et al. [13] grafted the medial basal hypothalamus from new born rats into the third ventricle of 21- to 30-month-old constant estrous Wistar rats. Three weeks after transplantation, recipients of hypothalamic transplants showed a significant increase in ovarian weight and some ovaries contained healthy-appearing corpora lutea and follicles of varying sizes. Rogers et al. [12] also reported that progressive changes of vaginal cyclicity during aging can be halted and partially reserved by implanting fetal medial preoptic area into the third ventricle of aged female rats. By implanting female fetal anterior hypothalamus into both sides of preoptic areas of hypothalamus in 16- to 18-month-old constant-estrus female rats, we found that 8 out of 9 old females reinitiated estrous cycles 1 month after transplantation. One remained in constant-estrus stage (table II) [Huang et al., unpubl. data]. However, the estrous cycles are irregular, most of them are prolonged estrous stages. None of the cerebral-cortex-grafted and intact controls resumed estrous cycles. Only 1 female had a prolonged diestrous stage during the experimental period. The ovarian and body weights are not different between the experimental and control groups. No new corpora lutea were observed in the ovaries. It is apparent that the resumed estrous cycles are anovulatory cycles.

Table II. Effect of fetal hypothalamic transplants on the vaginal cyclicity and ovaries in old constant-estrus female rats

Groups and number of animals	Average body weight, g	Average ovary weight mg/100 g body weight	Vaginal cyclicity
Hypothalamus graft (n = 9)	306.6 ± 37.3	20.5 ± 2.5	IC (8) CE (1)
Controls			
Intact (n = 4)	286.5 ± 22.9	18.5 ± 3.1	CE (4)
Brain cortex graft (n = 8)	299.6 ± 26.7	18.6 ± 2.4	CE (7) PD (1)

The grafts were transplanted into both sides of preoptic area. The values are given as means ± SD. The figures in parentheses indicate the number of rats. IC = Irregular cycle; CE = constant estrus; PD = prolonged diestrus [Huang et al., unpubl. data].

Discussion

The experimental studies reported here, as well as reports by Matsumoto et al. [13] and Rogers et al. [12] indicate that fetal and neonatal hypothalamic transplant can survive, develop and differentiate in the brain of aged host. Furthermore, it also can rejuvenate the neuroendocrine and reproductive function of the aged recipients. The impotent old male rats can respond to graft of fetal hypothalamic tissue with increased LH and testosterone release, and restoration of sexual function and fertility. Reinitiation of estrous cycles can also be induced by the transplant of hypothalamic tissue in old constant-estrous female rats. As mentioned in the introduction, many studies have demonstrated that the decline of reproductive function in rats during aging is largely due to an alteration of hypothalamic function. This alteration may be related to the decrease in hypothalamic catecholamines and increase in serotonin concentration and metabolism, which could account for the reduced secretions of LHRH and gonadotropins and increased secretion of prolactin in old rats. Increased neuroendocrine and reproductive function in old rats resulting from the fetal hypothalamic transplant indicates that deteriorating function of aged hypothalamic tissue can be restored. The fetal neural tissue which was grafted into the brain of aged hosts contained the embryonic neurons of LHRH, biogenic amines, other neurotransmitters and hormone-releasing factors. It can survive and apparently affect the aged host hypothalamus.

Recently, we have found an increase in hypothalamic catecholamine activities, and a decreased release of prolactin in the aged male rats with successful fetal hypothalamic grafts [unpubl. data]. These suggest that fetal hypothalamic transplants can produce catecholamines which functionally affect host brain, which in turn may stimulate the host hypothalamus to synthesize LHRH and decrease release of prolactin and increase gonadal function. Fetal or newborn hypothalamic tissues can differentiate and have LHRH activity when transplanted into the third ventricle of old constant-estrus female rats. The ovarian function and estrous cycles of the aged host can be partially resumed by the transplant [12, 13].

Since sexual behavior is the product of a combination of neuroendocrine control and several behavior elements, the decline of sexual function in old animals is not a simple function of reduced sex hormones. Thus, there are several possibilities to explain the restoration of sexual function and fertility by fetal hypothalamic graft in impotent aged male rats. The first possibility is that the neural graft can stimulate the aged host to secrete more gonadotropins and testosterone. The second possibility is that the increased activities of hypothalamic catecholamines and LHRH in the aged host may lower the threshold to testosterone in the neural sexual behavior mechanism. In a longitudinal study of aging rats, decline in the sexual behavior was not correlated with the change in testosterone level. Sexual behavior as a whole, and sexual motivation in particular, has not been shown to be a single factor of a reduced testosterone level [14]. LHRH has a facilitatory effect on male sexual behavior in rats with low testosterone levels, which could become limiting when testosterone decreases in aging [15]. LHRH is also capable of stimulating sexual arousal in rats by intraventricular injection of a subliminal dose [16]. The third possibility is the inhibition of prolactin release by the hypothalamic graft. Prolactin, which has an inhibitory effect on sexual behavior, is elevated in both male and female aged rats [4, 17, 18]. We have reported that suppression of prolactin release by injection of *L*-dopa, a precursor of catecholamines, can enhance the release of gonadotropins and reinitiate estrous cycles in old female rats [8]. Taken all together, rejuvenation of neuroendocrine function and restoration of reproductive function in aged rats by transplanting fetal hypothalamic tissue is not simply the administration of certain hormones or drugs which prompts acute stimulation of neuroendocrine system. Rather it seems to be akin to the mechanism proposed by Rogers et al. [12] in which the brain transplant can in many ways be considered as an ultimate implantable minipump. The transplants are self-maintaining and chronically release only the most 'natural' substances. They are limited neither to a single substance nor to a single channel for delivery and they may be able to deliver the right neurotransmitters or hormones to the right neural targets, thereby enhancing efficacy and minimizing unwanted side effect.

References

1 Larsson, K.: Sexual activity in senile male rats. J. Geront. *13:* 136–139 (1958).

2 Gray, G.D.; Smith, E.R.; Dorsa, D.M.; Davidson, J.M.: Sexual behavior and testosterone in middle-aged male rats. Endocrinology *109:* 1597–1604 (1981).

3 Huang, H.H.; Simpkins, J.W.; Meites, J.: Hypothalamic norepinephrine (NE) and dopamine (DA) turnover and relation to LH, FSH and prolactin release in old female rat. Endocrinology, suppl. 100, p. 331 (1977).

4 Simpkins, J.W.; Mueller, G.P.; Huang, H.H.; Meites, J.: Evidence for depressed catecholamine and enhanced serotonin metabolism in aging male rats: possible relation to gonadotropin secretion. Endocrinology *100:* 1672–1678 (1977).

5 Demarest, K.T.; Riegle, G.D.; Moore, K.E.: Characteristics of dopaminergic neurons in the aged male rats. Neuroendocrinology *31:* 222–227 (1980).

6 Hsu, H.K.; Peng, M.T.: Hypothalamic neuron number of old female rats. Gerontology *24:* 434–440 (1978).

7 Sabel, B.A.; Stein, D.G.: Extensive loss of subcortical neurons in the aging rat brain. Expl. Neurol. *73:* 507–516 (1981).

8 Huang, H.H.; Marshall, S.; Meites, J.: Induction of estrous cycles in old noncyclic rats by progesterone, ACTH, ether stress or *L*-Dopa. Neuroendocrinology *20:* 434–440 (1976).

9 Meites, J.; Huang, H.H.; Simpkins, J.W.: Recent studies on neuroendocrine control of reproductive senescence in rats; in Schneider, The aging reproductive system, pp. 213–235 (Raven Press, New York, 1978).

10 Gage, F.H.; Dunnett, S.B.; Stenevi, U.; Bjorklund, A.: Aged rats: recovery of motor impairments by intrastriatal nigral grafts. Science 221: 966–969 (1983).

11 Gage, F.H.; Dunnett, S.B.; Bjorklund, A.: Spatial learning and motor deficits in aged rats. Neurobiol. Aging *5:* 43–48 (1984).

12 Rogers, J.; Hoffman, G.E.; Zornetzer, S.F.; Vale, W.W.: Hypothalamic grafts and neuroendocrine cascade theories of aging; in Sladek, Gash, Neural transplants: development and function, pp. 205–222 (Plenum Press, New York 1984).

13 Matsumoto, A.; Kobayashi, S.; Marlsami, S.; Arai, Y.: Recovery of declined ovarian function in aged female rats by transplantation of newborn hypothalamic tissue. Proc. Jap. Acad. *60:* 73–76 (1984).

14 Davidson, J.M.; Gray, G.D.; Smith, E.R.: The sexual psychoendocrinology of aging; in Meites, Neuroendocrinology of aging, pp. 221–258 (Plenum, New York 1983).

15 Moss, R.L.; Dudley, C.A.; Foreman, M.M.; McCann, S.M.: Synthetic LRF; potentiator of sexual behavior in the rat; in Motta, Crosignonni, Martini, Hypothalamic hormones, p. 269 (Academic Press, New York, 1975).

16 Dorsa, D.M.; Smith, E.R.: Facilitation of mounting behavior in male rats by intracranial injection of luteinizing hormone-releasing hormone. Regul. Pept. *1:* 147–155 (1980).
17 Huang, H.H.; Steger, R.W.; Sonntag, W.E.; Meites, J.: Positive feedback by ovarian hormones on prolactin and LH in old versus young female rats. Neurobiol. Aging *1:* 141–143 (1980).
18 Huang, H.H.; Marshall, S.; Meites, J.: Capacity of old versus young female rats to secrete LH, FSH and prolactin. Biol. Reprod. *14:* 538–543 (1976).
19 Huang, H.H.; Kissane, J.Q.; Hawrylewicz, E.J.: Restoration of sexual function and fertility by fetal hypothalamic transplant in impotent aged male rats. Neurobiol. Aging *8:* 465–472 (1987).

Dr. Henry H. Huang, Department of Research, Mercy Hospital and Medical Center, Stevenson Expressway at King Drive, Chicago, IL 60616 (USA)

Subject Index